"*Aging Fabulously?* I can re[late], but then my hair turned s[ilver at] the beginning. Adams, Clyl[burn, and Lovely came] together and penned a wonderful devotional for those of us reaching for the doorbell or already through the door of senior sisterhood. I chuckled and even shed a few tears as I read through these sweet, touch-the-heart devotions. They opened my heart to the fact that aging is just a sweet step, and doing it fabulously means I've taken the Master's hand and pulled him into my heart. *Aging Fabulously - 52 Devotions Sure to Give You a Faith-Lift* is a book every woman, young or golden, needs on their nightstand."

—**Cindy K. Sproles**
Best-selling, award-winning author of
Meet Me Where I Am, Lord - 90 Days to Know Him Better
and *This is Where It Ends.*

"Growing old isn't for the faint of heart, they say – but authors Adams, Clyburn, and Lovely would rather say aging can be fabulous, fun, fancy, and faith-filled! Through the pages of 52 devotions, readers will giggle some, belly-laugh often, shed a tear or two, nod in agreement and say, "I know that's right," and embellish the heart with relevant verses from God's Word to walk into the 50s and beyond with hope, encouragement, and inspiration. Link arms with the authors of *Aging Fabulously* and march into the beautiful season of life God's ordained just for you!"

—**Julie Lavender**
Author of *Strength for All Seasons: A Mom's Devotional
of Powerful Verses and Prayers* and
Children's Bible Stories for Bedtime,
and *365 Ways to Love Your Child:
Turning Little Moments into Lasting Memories,*

"My mother taught me about skin care and healthcare, even at a young age, but my grandmother taught me the most important lesson of all when it comes to aging. One afternoon, while rocking lazily in two of the front porch rockers of her gracious Southern home, Grandmother asked, 'Darling, what do you want to be when you grow up?' Without blinking, I answered, 'I want to grow up to be like you,' I said. 'A sweet old lady.' Grandmother didn't take these words as insult, but as an opportunity to teach my young heart and mind. 'Sweet *old* ladies,' she said, 'come from sweet *young* ladies.' Just as with my mother's teachings for skin care, my grandmother poured into my heart what I needed to know about the inner me. Being sweet was just the start. Now that I *am* a 'sweet old lady,' I can tell you that, as wonderful as it can be growing 'old,' nothing is as lovely as growing old with Christ ... and with good Christian friends who write devotionals like this one. *Aging Fabulously* will make you smile, laugh, and ponder ... which is one of the things we older chicks do best."

—**Eva Marie Everson**
CEO, Word Weavers International, Inc. and
Award-winning Author of many books including,
Our God is Bigger Than That! and *The Third Path*

"So you found a gray hair or two? Don't throw a pity party, instead celebrate your now with *Aging Fabulously* by devo authors Adams, Clyburn, and Lovely. Enjoy their personal stories, prayer, and sassy suggestions that will inspire and refuel you for your continuing journey into amazing."

—**Linda Evans Shepherd**
Award-winning author of 38 books,
and founder of the Advanced Writers & Speakers Association

"With humor, spiritual insights, and practical tips, Adams, Clyburn, and Lovely offer confidence for the season of life women fear most. *Aging Fabulously* invites readers to face seniority with grace and power. Each devotion relates to our common struggles and shares insights to help us develop the resilience found only in the timelessness of our faith. Daily sips of inspiration from these wise, author sisters offer the renewing motivation women need to thrive in our final quarter of life. I highly recommend *Aging Fabulously* as a recurring dose of much-needed assurance for women over forty."

—**Tina Yeager**, LMHC
Award-winning author, emotional health coach,
Flourish-Meant Podcast host,
Flourish Today radio show host, and speaker

Michelle Medlock Adams
Connie Clyburn
Cynthia A. Lovely

aging fabulously

52 Devotions Sure to Give You a Faith-Lift

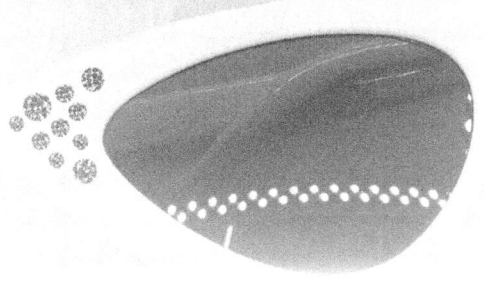

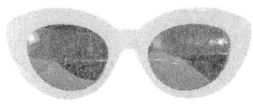

aging fabulously

52 Devotions Sure to Give You a Faith-Lift

Michelle Medlock Adams
Connie Clyburn
Cynthia A. Lovely

Bold Vision Books
PO Box 2011
Friendswood, TX 77549

Copyright © Michelle Medlock Adams, Connie Clyburn, Cynthia A. Lovely 2023

ISBN 978-1-946708-94-6
Library of Congress Control Number

All rights reserved.
Published by Bold Vision Books, PO Box 2011, Friendswood, Texas 77549
www.boldvisionbooks.com

Published in association with literary agent Cyle Young Literary Elite
Cover Art by Amber Weigand-Buckley
Cover Design by Barefaced Creative Media
Interior design by WendyEL Creative.
Editor: Cherry McGregor

Published in the United States of America.

All rights reserved. No part of this publication may be reproduced, stored in a retrieval system, or transmitted in any form or by any means—electronic, mechanical, photocopy, recording, or any other—except for brief quotations in printed reviews, without the prior permission of the publisher.

Scripture quotations marked (NIV) are taken from the Holy Bible, New International Version®, NIV®. Copyright © 1973, 1978, 1984, 2011 by Biblica, Inc.™ Used by permission of Zondervan. All rights reserved worldwide. www.zondervan.com The "NIV" and "New International Version" are trademarks registered in the United States Patent and Trademark Office by Biblica, Inc.™

Scripture quotations marked AMP are taken from the Amplified® Bible, Copyright © 1954, 1958, 1962, 1964, 1965, 1987 by The Lockman Foundation
Used by permission." (www.Lockman.org)

Scripture quotations marked ESV are taken from The Holy Bible, English Standard Version® (ESV®) Copyright © 2001 by Crossway, a publishing ministry of Good News Publishers. All rights reserved. ESV Text Edition: 2007

Scripture quotations marked NKJV are taken from the New King James Version®. Copyright © 1982 by Thomas Nelson, Inc. Used by permission. All rights reserved.
Scripture quotations marked "KJV" are taken from the Holy Bible, King James Version, Cambridge, 1769.

Scripture quotations marked TPT are from The Passion Translation®. Copyright © 2017, 2018 by Passion & Fire Ministries, Inc. Used by permission. All rights reserved. ThePassionTranslation.com.

Scripture quotations marked NLT are taken from the Holy Bible, New Living Translation, copyright ©1996, 2004, 2007 by Tyndale House Foundation. Used by permission of Tyndale House Publishers, Inc., Carol Stream, Illinois 60188. All rights reserved.

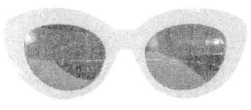

Dedications

Connie:
To my husband, Jeff, who "holds down the fort" while I work on my literary dreams. He's also been known to get creative at the last minute when I need a prop for a television appearance.

To my mom, Nancy, and my late father, Tom, who supported me no matter where my adventures led. I think mom would have brought food and supplies to me even if I'd traveled to the ends of the earth and dad would have been there, camera in hand, taking photos of the whole thing.

Cynthia:
In loving memory of my amazing mother who aged with wisdom, wit, compassion, and an unending love for Jesus, extending to all those around her.

Michelle:
Dedicated in memory of my feisty, faith-filled mama who aged fabulously and taught me to love Jesus and live every day to the fullest.

Contents

	introduction	11
1	joining the senior club	13
2	silver thread	17
3	big hair, don't care	21
4	beyond the filter	25
5	i shoulda' been a cowgirl	29
6	radiant and relevant	33
7	popcorn and a movie	37
8	what's in a name?	41
9	bugs be gone	45
10	i get by with a little help from my friends	49
11	friends forever	53
12	superior moments	57
13	undistracted	61
14	stand strong	65
15	the golden years	69
16	here's to your health	73
17	i can see clearly now	77
18	mirror reflection	81
19	sweet speech & stronger bones	85
20	the spiritual senior special	89
21	all things subject to change	93
22	seeking the kingdom	97
23	faith at any age	101
24	root of bitterness	107
25	a special place of prayer	111
26	sometimes i'm up, sometimes i'm down	115
27	growing up gracefully	119

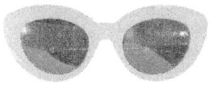

28	moving on	123
29	don't be a qsw	127
30	the poetry of marriage	131
31	sunset and strife	135
32	kid stuff 101	139
33	memory lane of thanks	143
34	surprise! when life delivers the unexpected	147
35	life is better with laughter	151
36	a season of harvest	155
37	five finger life	159
38	victorious living	163
39	the final category	167
40	scrooge thieves	171
41	defeating giants	175
42	rejoice in life	179
43	naptime	183
44	dwell and rest	187
45	lullaby and good night	191
46	the mountains are calling	195
47	never too late	199
48	he notices	203
49	lifetime achievements	207
50	if you need me, i'll be in the antique store	211
51	legacy of love	215
52	god's treasure	219

acknowledgments 223
about the authors 225

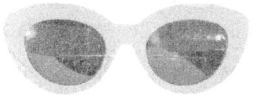

introduction

Someone once said, "Age is simply the number of years the world has been enjoying you." Love that quote. You see, many books for people over 50 are so serious and lackluster that you'd think aging is the worst thing that could happen to you. Not so. Truly, it's the best thing that could happen to you because it means you're still alive. You're still here for a reason. You've got more to do on this earth. And that's exactly why we wrote this book—to celebrate the privilege of getting older and to change the old stereotype of what *older* actually means.

We—Michelle, Connie, and Cynthia,—are three gal pals who have joined efforts to produce relevant and inspiring entries that Gen X'rs and Boomers alike will enjoy. We wrote every word with you in mind. We know what you're facing. We understand the fears you might have. And we totally get both the beauty and aggravation of aging—because we are right there with you.

From celebrating sisterhood to pursuing new adventures, this devotional is designed to cheer your heart with compassion and comradery. We have structured it with a key verse at the top of each entry, the devotion itself, a prayer, and a section called "Sassy Suggestions" which features additional practical information we thought you might enjoy. With 52 entries, you can do one each week and ponder the truths from that devotion for seven days, or you can read one each day if you prefer. We encourage you to hunker down in your favorite chair, grab your cup of coffee or hot chocolate, and ready your heart for what God wants to share with you. Also, you might want to use a designated journal and make notes and answer the questions we ask throughout this devotional. But more than anything, we want you to enjoy this journey with us.

We want you to know that you are more than just a number, and so are we. We are all savvy, sassy, mature women who have gained wisdom (and yes, a few wrinkles) over the years, and it's time we celebrate who we are and whose we are.

We pray these devotions make you laugh, cry, ponder, affirm, giggle and finally to resolve in your heart and mind that aging doesn't have to be feared, it can be fabulous—just like you.

Your Faith-Lift awaits ...

1

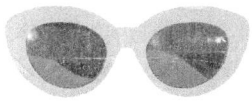

Very truly I tell you, whoever hears my word and believes him who sent me has eternal life and will not be judged but has crossed over from death to life (John 5:24 NIV).

joining the senior club

Michelle Medlock Adams

The other day as I finished my shopping, I hopped into the checkout line. When it was finally my turn, I quickly placed my items on the counter, when the salesclerk innocently asked, "Are you a senior? On Wednesdays, our senior club members get an extra 20 percent discount."

Let me tell you, if looks could kill, that perky woman would've been belly up. I quickly informed her I did *not* qualify for the senior discount. She smirked and continued ringing up my items.

I walked out of that store with a bit of embarrassment churning in the pit of my stomach. Nothing humbles you quite like being told out of the blue, "Hey, you look old, but you *do* qualify for a discount, so there's that." Even if I *were* old enough to join the *senior club*, I don't know that I'd want to join. Who enjoys announcing, "I'd like the senior discount, please," in front of everyone in the store?

But that retail encounter started me thinking. The one nice perk about senior memberships is you don't need to do anything special to join. You don't need to pay an annual membership fee or meet a long list of requirements. The store covers the costs and offers discounts and perks just for showing up as you are—even if *as you are* involves bifocal glasses and every anti-wrinkle product known to man. All you have to do in order to qualify is be who you are.

There's another club that operates in much the same way—the *Christian Club*. We qualify to be in the Christian Club just by showing up as we are. Jesus has covered the cost and it was a big price to pay. He faced the pain of death on a cross so that we could enjoy freedom from sin and eternal life in union with the Father. All we need to do is accept his offer—repent of our sins and ask him to be the Lord of our lives—and we're part of the family.

Accepting that offer changes everything. When you decide, *I believe Jesus died and rose from the grave; I believe he has the power to forgive my sinful nature and I accept the grace he has extended to me,* it frees you from living life in shame. It frees you from the fear of death. The decision gives you a friend you can depend on and it gives your life purpose, peace, and hope.

Now, that's not to say that life in the Christian Club is always full of discounts and perks. Even after you accept Jesus as your Lord and Savior, life can still be hard. Doubt might creep into your mind, whispering, *Maybe that offer you accepted in your heart is just too good to be true.*

But hear this, friend—the Lord is working, even when you can't see it. When bad situations happen, from something as trivial as losing your car keys to something as serious as a scary diagnosis, God will go through them with you. And the Word tells us in Romans 8:28 that God works all things together for good for those who love the Lord.

If you haven't ever accepted Jesus as your Lord and Savior—the greatest offer of all time—I invite you to ponder it in your heart now. Just say yes to the forgiveness, love, and new life that Jesus offers, and start enjoying all the benefits that come with this Christian Club membership. So much better than any senior discount. I promise.

prayer:

Dear Lord, Thank you for sending your Son to earth to save us from sin and offer us eternal life with you. I am so grateful. Thank you, Lord. I accept with an open heart, and I give my whole life to you. In Jesus' name. Amen.

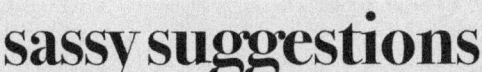

sassy suggestions

» Spend some time meditating on what it really means to be in the Christian Club. What costs did Jesus cover? What benefits come with membership in the family of God? There are so many. Psalm 68:19 even confirms it. "Blessed be the Lord, who daily loadeth us with benefits, even the God of our salvation" (KJV).

» The next time someone offers you a senior discount—whether you accept or decline—do it with a smile.

2

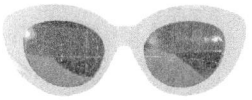

Gray hair is a crown of splendor; it is attained in the way of righteousness (Proverbs 16:31 NIV).

silver thread

Cynthia A. Lovely

do you remember the day you found it? It was like any other day with no warning of the rude awakening that was to come.

You were going about the day as usual, but somewhere along the way you glanced in the mirror. The light was just right and caught the single silver strand in your hair. What? You looked closer and tilted your head at all angles until you looked like a bobble-head doll. Yep, still there. It was a day of facing reality, the entrance into the world occupied by all those … older people.

Well, when it happened to me, I think I laughed. It was not one single strand, but a few small strands around my ears when I pulled my long hair back into a low braid. Wow, look at that. I wondered how it got there. How had I missed the first lonely strand and how soon would my entire head be covered in gray? I had to decide if this possibility disturbed me.

Honestly, I determined not to stress over it. Searching through scriptures, I found some interesting verses on gray hair. It is a crown of splendor. I like this phrase. Crowns are known to be a headdress for royalty. Read that again, please. Crowns symbolize authority and honor, worn by kings and queens. Since we are part of God's kingdom, it makes sense. And I don't know about you, but I like the title of Queen.

Researching further, we see gray hair is a crown of *splendor*. This word brings forth images of magnificence, grandeur, and elegance. Yes, yes, and yes. Gray hair is looking more attractive all the time. Reading on, we see this blessing is *attained in the way of righteousness*. Attained means we are reaching for something, trying to accomplish, achieve, or gain with a purpose. So if we follow Jesus and walk in his path of righteousness, this may be a part of his blessing. Certainly places a whole new look at turning gray.

Personally, I have always looked up to older women with silvery hair who have an air of being stylish and graceful. Somehow, they wear the threads of wisdom well. And I believe they showcase wisdom gained through the years. If I am teased about turning gray, I remind others that I have earned every gray strand. Whether through troubles, sorrow, heartache or simply the pressures of life on earth, each touch of gray symbolizes my long journey.

I think of the silver being like medals of honor. This strand came about when I made a tough decision and left a stressful job for something better. A few others developed when dealing with difficult relationships and trying to live peacefully among friends and family. Newer touches of silver appeared after caregiving for my parents and helping them move to a new location and giving up their home of so many years.

Yes, I earned each thread of new color and I hope to wear the silvery touches well. It seems like more and more women are embracing the gray and turning it into a stylish and attractive choice. So, wear your crown, not with pride but with joy, for following the way of righteousness. And if you really can't accept it, that's fine, too. There are methods to work around it if you feel you must. As we grow older, we are free to make these decisions for ourselves. But for me and my hair, we will accept the color silver. I admit, silver sounds classier than the word gray.

When I hear the word silver, several images and descriptions come to mind: Silver is valuable, priceless, sparkling, elegant, alluring, classic, hi-tech, and modern. What do you think of when you hear this word? I recognize and value my silver threads.

prayer:

Dear Lord, we thank you for your crown of splendor. May we wear it humbly before you and showcase your beauty as we age in your wisdom and strength. In Jesus' name. Amen.

sassy suggestions:

» To gray or not to gray. This topic brings to light one of the physical changes women may face as they get older. Maybe that day of discovering a silver strand has already happened to you. And I imagine it brought about a multitude of thoughts along with the discovery.

» Physical appearance will change with each year. As we allow God to work on our attitude, we will realize we are and always will be God's beautiful creation. We should remind ourselves of this every time we look in a mirror.

» The challenge may be for us to avoid the trap of looking and feeling frumpy. Rather, let us pattern ourselves after older women who are lovely with a rare combination of inner beauty and calmness shining through, along with tasteful choices in dress, hairstyles, and accessories.

» I look up to older women with carefully coiffed silver hair, maybe woven in a beautiful coronet, who dress with elegance and grace in styles that are classic. Let's dress fashionably without trying to be 25 again.

» As we take time to present a fresh appearance, we can turn to what truly matters—our inner beauty. Inner beauty is the love of God shining through our countenance and our mannerisms. This holy glow is present when we have spent time with Jesus, growing older in the beauty of his holiness.

3

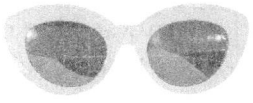

It is because of the Lord's lovingkindness that we are not consumed; Because His (tender) compassions never fail (Lamentations 3:22 AMP).

big hair, don't care

Connie Clyburn

The higher the hair, the closer to Jesus. If that's true, then Jesus and I are BFFs, for sure. Big hair because, after all the hair styles stops I've made through the years, it seems I have arrived back in Big Hair Town. It's big and wavy at present because I've concluded that I should stop trying to contain it and just let it do what it wants. My hair is like that unruly child in the toy aisle throwing a fit until its parent gives in and lets it do what it wants.

An old friend I run into now and then never fails to comment about my constantly changing hairdos. I don't try to keep up with every changing wind of style, but I do get bored with my hair. I think that's how I take a walk on the wild side—with a new do. I don't get tattoos, so I guess the next best thing is changing my hair (not knocking tattoos, it's just not for me).

I get the big hair gene from both sides of my family. My paternal grandmother had so much hair even at age 86 that I could hardly find the ends to help her get it all up in curlers. I also remember, as a child, sitting in the kitchen watching my mom and her sisters put Toni perms in each other's hair. Little pink plastic rollers and smelly perm solution transformed their semi wavy hair into tight springy curls that were much easier to manage in the summer heat while hoeing weeds in the garden and breaking beans on the porch. My mother set her sights on my hair and worked her curling magic until the day I managed to break free from her hairdo hacienda. Her motto was *Give everyone a perm, achieve world peace.*

The only problem—my heavy, thick hair, under the spell of perm solution, expands. Though mom never figured out that was a bad thing, I realized over the years the permed look was not a good one for me. It made for lots of interesting school photos of me that still make me gasp and laugh out loud. Oh my. My heart followed the hair fads wherever they led. I've made the circle and returned to the curly hair look after going through the straight hair stage, short hair, and the pixie haircut. My big hair now does its own thing. I've stopped trying to contain it with straight irons and smoothing spray. After spending a small fortune over the years, I've figured out my hair is going to do what it wants, no matter what goop I use to tame it.

My life has been like a tale of hairdos. College days and summer jobs took me through my various life stages. Some I'd just as soon forget, and others left me with good friends who have kept in touch. I look back and see where God has guided me and my hair through situations and away from those where I didn't need to go. He has been constant in my life, always nearby. I remember a brief time of uncertainty in college, where he sent just the right person to help guide me back on the right path. It was at that moment that he shook me back to reality.

He allows me to be myself with gentle nudges of his love. Knowing he has stayed close to me throughout my life keeps me constantly following him. The years leading to where I am now show me that God has loved me through my life—hairdos and all. I'm sure my hair style choices have amused him too. He never abandoned me when I felt unsure. My questions never caused him to run out the door, like I did when the Toni perm solution got too strong and stinky.

The latest fads can look all shiny and new, but quickly fade, leaving us looking to freshen ourselves up again. The good news is God never changes with the fads. His way never goes out of style. He is constant through every change we go through—the good and the bad. Like hairdos, life ebbs and flows, but his way and his Word remain the same.

prayer:

Dear Lord, Thank you for loving me through my life changes, even when I've failed like a bad perm. You've remained constantly devoted to me. You held on to me even when I decided to follow crazy fads that went nowhere. I love you, Jesus. I'm yours, big hair and all, for eternity. In Jesus' name. Amen.

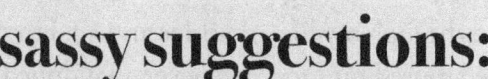

sassy suggestions:

» **Perms will eventually come unraveled, but establishing yourself in God's Word will ensure your life doesn't.**

» **Though friends and family have the best intentions, we make our own choices in life. Listening to sound advice is important, but in the end, we must find out what the Word has to say about it, pray, and then make up our own minds.**

» **God loves us through our ups and downs. His Word says he will never leave nor forsake his children.**

» **Just because everyone is participating in the latest fad doesn't mean it's the right choice for you.**

» **Be who God made you to be. You are unique, hair and all, and God has you on a certain path for his purposes.**

4

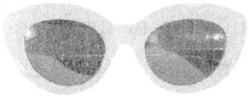

But the Lord said to Samuel, 'Do not look on his appearance or on the height of his stature, because I have rejected him. For the Lord sees not as man sees: man looks on the outward appearance, but the Lord looks on the heart (1 Samuel 16:7 ESV).

beyond the filter

Michelle Medlock Adams

Have you ever been talking to someone you assumed was *waaay* older than you, only to learn the person was your age? Or—even worse—the person was actually younger than you? That's when the thought hits you ... *Wait, do I look that old?*

After years of seeing yourself in the mirror every day, you assume nothing has changed in the past year, or five, or ten. It's like the best Instagram filter ever. But then, when we look at those around us, we become a bit more critical. *It's those other people who look and act old—certainly I could never be that way.* Over time, I think we see ourselves through very forgiving eyes. Or maybe, it's that our eyesight has become so blurry, we truly think we look the same. I admit it. I was guilty of this.

That is, until I started studying my reflection in one of those magnification mirrors. Yikes! That's when it all becomes clear—a new forehead wrinkle, a few more smile lines, and are those age spots on my cheek? Suddenly, I think thoughts like, *Should I get that miracle face serum I've been seeing on social media? Or maybe I should start consuming that collagen drink I read about in that beauty magazine?*

Magnification mirrors make it easy to become critical of ourselves.

But I have some good news for you. God doesn't see us that way. He looks past everything on the outside and looks right at our hearts. That's what matters to him. He sees the very best in us.

And it gets even better than that. Jesus created his own filter for us. When Jesus gave his life on the cross and conquered death, he made it so all the ugly stuff could be wiped off of our hearts. The Father doesn't have to look at us and see us coated in sin. The Jesus filter doesn't just cover up blemishes; it erases them for good.

When you find it difficult to look past your inner flaws—whether it's a streak of selfishness or a jealous spirit—you can approach God boldly, knowing that Jesus already paid the price for your sin, and that God's mercies are new every single morning. All you have to do is ask God to forgive you, and he will.

When you become focused on the flaws of others, try to see them through God's eyes. Remember the forgiveness you have received through Jesus, and offer that same grace—after all, we're told in scripture to forgive one another as God has forgiven us. It's time to look at ourselves and others through the Jesus filter.

Now, back to those external reminders that we're getting older … I get it. The thought of looking old can sometimes feel daunting. It's hard when you feel the millennials looking at you like you're ancient or when a store clerk assumes you're old enough to get the senior discount, or when a new age spot pops up overnight. But in the end, God's opinion is the only one that matters. I'd much rather be beautiful in God's eyes than get too wrapped up in what everyone else thinks. Wouldn't you? Full disclosure—I bought that beauty serum, and it truly is like "Botox in a bottle."

prayer:

Dear Lord, Thank you for looking at me with such love, even when I feel like I'm a hot mess half of the time. Lord, help me focus more on my inner beauty. Transform me, Lord. Make me more like you. I ask you to forgive me for the ugly things in my heart and to replace them with your perfect love.
In Jesus' name. Amen.

sassy suggestions:

» **Do a heart check. Is there anything ugly in there that needs to be fixed? Pray for help identifying and mending anything that needs attention.**

» **Find something nice to say about every person you encounter today. Of course, you should be sincere, but I bet you can find something positive about everyone you see.**

5

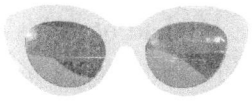

Therefore become imitators of God (copy Him and follow His example), as well-beloved children (imitate their father)
(Ephesians 5:1 AMP).

i shoulda' been a cowgirl

Connie Clyburn

I want to ride the prairie, herd cows, and eat beans from a can. That idea sounds good until I realize that includes ... actually riding the prairie in the hot sun, herding smelly cows all day, and eating cold beans from a can. Still, the old westerns are some of my favorites—television, movies, and books use fact mingled with fiction to tell stories of the American cowboy, Native Americans, and the Wild West. I love it all. I'm pretty sure I got it from my dad. He loved all things western. I think he secretly wanted to live on the Ponderosa, made famous on the *Bonanza* television show, and ride the prairie.

I grew to appreciate my dad's love for westerns as I got older. The younger me kept up with other goings on in the world as I went through college and then became a newspaper reporter. Along the way, though, I started to resemble my dad more and more. I developed an interest in what had been his hobbies. I love capturing images with my camera and my phone camera. I find myself wishing I'd kept all his photography equipment we sold after my dad died. I can see some of my dad's ways in me—his gentle nature, his love of a good story, and eating at steakhouses. Old wagon wheels, big belt buckles, CB handles, and the Chuck Wagon Gang (singing group) all remind me of him. Not that I'm embracing all of them, but memories of my old dad and a good cup of coffee give me the warm fuzzies. That's another trait—my dad loved coffee and I didn't care for it until a few years ago.

As much as I love my dad and see some of his characteristics in me, I want even more to be like my heavenly Father (my earthly dad would heartily approve). I observe little children as they watch their fathers, trying to imitate every action. They hold on to their dad's hand and take gigantic kid-sized steps along with his big adult steps. Watch a little one as it puts its tiny feet into dad's big shoes and then tries walking in those oversized shoes. It stumbles and fumbles around because the shoes are much too big. The child is not quite ready for adult shoes. When I first began following God, I stumbled around until I started growing in my Christian walk, learning more and more about my heavenly Father. As I grew from one stage to the next, I became more and more like him.

All of us are like that. We grow in God's Word and learn how to imitate our heavenly Father as we study and get deep into the Word. This is where he speaks to us, showing us how to imitate him. We learn how to be led by the Holy Spirit and listen to his still, small voice. It may seem like slow going at first, just like the little kid trying to walk in its father's shoes, but the more we follow in his footsteps, the more we will start to resemble him. If you get stuck, just ask the Lord to open and increase your understanding of his Word. He's waiting to help.

You may wonder how you could ever imitate God. After all, he is God, Creator of all, Omnipotent Father. There's the key—he is our Father God. You are his well-beloved child who, just like an earthly child, longs to be just like his or her father. It's not hard. Watch your heavenly Father, see how he works, listen to his Word being taught and read what he says in it.

During his earthly ministry, Jesus said that he only did what his Father God told him to do. "So Jesus answered them by saying, 'I assure you *and* most solemnly say to you, the Son can do nothing of Himself (of His own accord) unless it is something He sees the Father doing; for whatever things the Father does, the Son (in His turn) also does in the same way" (John 5:19 AMP).

Jesus watched and listened to his Father, exemplifying God's will for us as we live on the earth. Studying Jesus' earthly ministry as told in the Gospels will also help us grow as well-beloved children imitating their Father.

prayer:

Dear Lord, I want to be more like you every day. Thank you for filling me with your Holy Spirit, who leads and guides me in your paths. I love you. In Jesus' name. Amen.

sassy suggestions:

» Jesus said he only did what his Father God told him to do. Study the Gospels and list all the miracles Jesus performed. Pay special attention to the words he spoke as he carried out his Father's will.

» Make a list of ways to imitate God on the earth and think of activities that exemplify his love for others.

» Host a Bible study with friends. Make it a cozy and fun time with coffee served in brightly colored mugs, along with yummy cookies to munch as you discuss God's Word.

» Make flash cards displaying verses to post around in your home—no matter which room you're in, you'll have God's Word there to remind you that you are his child.

» Make fun gift tags or cards to include with gifts for friends and family, to help encourage them in their walk as well-beloved children imitating their heavenly Father.

6

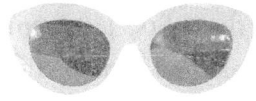

Older women likewise are to be reverent in behavior, not slanderers or slaves to much wine. They are to teach what is good, and so train the young women to love their husbands and children …
(Titus 2:3-4 ESV).

radiant and relevant

Cynthia A. Lovely

The phrase older women jumped out at me. I glanced around to see if anyone was watching. No, it was safe to read on and admit the truth—I qualified for this verse. My take on this scripture is I need to behave (working on that part) not slander or gossip about anyone (yes!) and avoid much wine (not a problem.) Good to go—simple instructions.

The verse continues on with advice on teaching the younger women all that is good, training them to love their husbands and their children. The work at home part probably looked very different back then but fits right in with today's season of Covid.

Some of the other words and imagery here may bring to mind an old-fashioned picture to which we may find hard to relate. However, there must be a way to connect with our present society and the current generation. We want to be relevant to the younger women in our church or social circles.

While pondering these thoughts, I remembered a beautiful blog post my friend Cathy Baker shared a while ago. She overheard a conversation at a coffee shop between a younger girl and an older woman. "Our generation needs women like you to pour into us." This statement from the younger woman stuck in Cathy's mind and helped her move forward when the opportunity arose to host a small gathering at her home. Most in the group were young college girls.

My friend related how she struggled with her emotions before the initial meeting. Feelings of excitement and anticipation battled against feelings of insecurity and nervousness. Her heart's desire was to affect these young women and be relevant. She had doubts about what she had to offer them besides freshly baked chocolate chip cookies—well, that's a great start. She pushed past the negativity when the girls began filing through her back door. In her words, "I did what any good southerner would do—I hugged the puddin' out of them."

They enjoyed a relaxed evening of fellowship, getting to know one another. And from that initial meeting, Cathy invited them to a special tea party. She went all out preparing for these women, determined to make it memorable. She used treasured china, a large pedestal platter filled with vanilla doozies wrapped in sprinkles, along with scones, sandwiches and tea. Cathy passed around a basket filled with hearts, one side gold and the other side paper. There was a handwritten verse on each one describing God's love. They ended the evening lighting individual candles and sharing their verses aloud. Each young woman received a sweet gift; a small bag filled with a Starbucks gift card, wrapped gumballs and chocolate kisses.

When I read this blog post along with the photos of the tea event, I teared up. The faces of these young girls, radiant and aglow from the candlelight, expressed an appreciation for an evening of *feeling special and feeling loved.* Cathy related to them simply by loving them. And who wouldn't love the sweets, scones, chocolates, candlelight, and scriptures emphasizing God's love? My friend met them on a basic level of love and concern, moving past her own insecurities.

By stretching past her comfort zone, Cathy opened the door to minister to these ladies and potentially affect their lives and their walk with God. Extending love to them first, she may be able to influence their future decisions and yes, to "teach what is good and to train the young women."

As older women, we have much to offer the younger girls among us. Through years of experience, making our own mistakes and learning wisdom along the way, we can help them avoid some of our own stumbling blocks and to grow in Christ. Cathy moved on after this event and created an online community, "Creative Pauses," and she continues to minister to others. But it started with one simple meeting. Small steps, moving forward. As God directs you, start to connect with the younger generation and watch what God will do.

prayer:

*Lord Jesus, help us see
the young women around us in this confusing and
troubled world, and to be brave enough to reach out to
them. Show us how to be loving and
kind and to affect this new generation.
In Jesus' name. Amen.*

sassy suggestions:

» Is there a young person you have noticed who seems troubled or looks like they need a friend? You may be the one to minister to a single lonely gal who needs to know someone cares for her.

» If you aren't a social butterfly and feel a bit awkward, think back to how you felt at their age. We have years of experience to pull from and once we get past the initial hesitation and realize the great need before us, we usually forget about ourselves.

» Try something simple, like sending a thoughtful card. Begin easy conversations. Move on to texting an encouraging scripture. Lead up to a phone call. You may be surprised how the Lord takes these little efforts to lead into his grand scheme and overall picture.

» If you are more like my sweet friend, open your home and your heart to these precious young people. And remember, even my more extroverted friend still had her own struggles with reaching past her comfort zone.

» No matter your personality, God is able to use your strengths and skills to make a difference to the young women in your life. Step out and reach out.

7

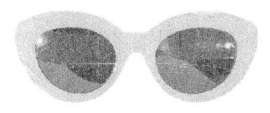

The thief comes only in order to steal kill and destroy. I came that they may have and enjoy life, and have it in abundance (to the full, till it overflows) (John 10:10 AMP).

popcorn and a movie

Connie Clyburn

The world outside my picture window promises fun times with good food and great friends. Soon, I'll sail down our long gravel driveway and turn toward the bright lights of the big city to meet up with my foodie group of besties. Or not.

I look at my boxer, Mary Grace, all curled up in a comfy heap on the bed, and I want to pop some popcorn, turn on a movie, and snuggle with her instead of going out. I love my friends and have fun getting together with them. Really, I do. Eating great food and shopping till I drop are two of my favorite activities. I lean on a pile of clothing lying in a big heap in my walk-in closet and ponder when this change in me occurred. I also realize that, should a tornado ever approach the house, we could seriously tunnel under all the stuff in my closet and be safe as bugs in a rolled-up rug. But I digress.

Weekend plans with friends are great—until you have to put on clothes and leave the house. I'm all *woo hoo* while discussing plans to go out for dinner. Then reality sets in when I realize I'll have to get off the couch and put on real clothes. I go to my cluttered closet and dig through shirts and pants I should have given away long ago. I grab something and pull on it, hoping I don't start an avalanche (true story). The soft and slightly faded lounging pants I've had on all day are really comfy. Do I dare wear them out in public? Could I stroll into the Cracker Barrel in these? I'm pretty sure someone has already blazed that trail before me.

I can go from being excited about making plans to wanting to stay home and watch a movie faster than you can say, "Party of eight". But I decide I can't let myself start drifting away from my people. I've seen some of my loved one's trade time socializing with the community for solitude that quickly becomes loneliness. It's sad because the world keeps turning and going on without them. I don't want to be one who ends up peering out through closed blinds at the world going on outside but never getting involved. I plan to be out there. I want to honor Jesus by staying active and involved.

One way I enjoy life to the fullest is by being part of the worship team at my church. There have been many times along the way that I've considered stepping aside. Every birthday reminds me I'm not a youngster. Then I remember I'm blessed with the ability to sing the harmonies that I love so much. God has given me this ability to use in leading his people into worship. I don't take that lightly. I can't decide on a whim that I no longer want to participate due to my age or any other reason. I repent of my attitude and decide to remain involved as long as that's where he wants me serving.

God has charged us all with certain duties that have no expiration date as long as we're on this side of the daisies. He's also equipped us with gifts and talents to accomplish them. It's up to us to walk in the abundant life Jesus has provided. Anything less would be failing to do what the Word says. I don't want to cooperate with the enemy's plans. Jesus paid an enormous price to give us abundant life so that we can enjoy this earthly walk as we carry out his Word.

Perhaps you want to do the same, but you're not sure how. Start by simply thanking God for your life. Then ask him to show you what your part is. Living abundantly has as much to do with a mindset as it does with having physical *things*. You can live in the grandest house on the block and not be living in abundance if your mind is set on lack. It doesn't matter what our bank account shows or even if our cabinets are full, experiencing a truly abundant life is trusting God no matter what our circumstances look like. Living abundantly is knowing that God is on our side. It's experiencing his love day after day, as he wakes us up each morning, bidding us to spend time with him. It's a decision he allows us to make. I choose to live in joy and overflow. How about you?

prayer:

*Dear Lord, Thank you for my life.
I will honor you every day, determined to walk in joy
and the other wonderful gifts you've given me.
There's no time to stay in the doldrums,
allowing the enemy to steal from me.
In Jesus' name. Amen.*

sassy suggestions:

» **Choose life.** Make it your purpose to live to the fullest each day, finding joy in everything you do.

» **Encourage others.** Find people who may not be living in abundant life and share with them how you have overcome the enemy's plan to keep you down in the dumps.

» **Sing it out.** It doesn't matter if your voice draws birds to sing along or howls from the neighbor's dog, sing praises to Jesus. Praising him will lift you up above any bad circumstances.

» **Movie night.** Invite your friends over for snacks and a movie. You get to spend time with your favorite people, and you get to stay home. Win-win.

» **Volunteer.** Helping others will put a spring in your step and help you find the joy of living.

8

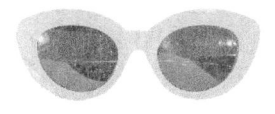

*A good name is to be chosen rather than great riches,
and favor is better than silver or gold
(Proverbs 22:1 ESV).*

what's in a name?

Michelle Medlock Adams

From the moment I found out our oldest daughter Abby was expecting our first grandchild, I began *trying out* grandma names. At only 47, I didn't feel like a grandmother—too formal. I also didn't feel like a Mamaw—that's what my mom had been called before she went to heaven. And I definitely didn't feel like a Nana—that was my mother-in-law's chosen grandma name, and it was the name of the big dog in Peter Pan, so there's that. I did a little research into other possible grandma names. I especially liked Mimi, but my sister Martie had already claimed that one. And I kind of liked the name *Glamma*, which a lady in my Zumba class explained was short for a glamorous grandma; however, that seemed like a lot to live up to, and I certainly wasn't glamorous all the time. So Glamma was also a no. And then I came across the grandma name, Gigi. I tried it on, and it just seemed to fit. And bonus—it's easy to find cute T-shirts and jewelry with the name Gigi proudly displayed. My favorite tank says, "In a world of grandmas, be a Gigi."

Names are important, whether we are choosing a grandma name for ourselves or naming our children or fur babies. Think back ... how did you come up with the names you gave to your kiddos? Often, we choose the name of a favorite relative or a sound biblical name, such as Matthew, Paul, Mary, or Mark. Other times, we simply select a name that flows well with our last name, which is what we did when we chose *Abby* and *Ally* for our daughters' names. Abby Adams and Ally Adams rolled off the tongue beautifully. Still, other parents name their children after favorite sports figures or celebrities or even seasons. When my sister had her youngest daughter on the last day of autumn, she decided to name her *Autumn* to signify that special day for all eternity.

And as important as names are in today's world, they were even more significant in bible times. Names back then were often chosen to reveal something specific about that person. Remember when God changed Abram's name? He went from Abram which meant *high father* to Abraham because it meant *father of many nations*. That name was given to Abraham to remind him and everyone who called him Abraham that he would one day be the father of many nations. It meant something. Every time someone said his name, it reminded Abraham of his destiny.

The many names found throughout the Bible reveal God's identity and character. The names of God are like miniature pictures and promises of who God is. Each of his mighty names reveals his very essence and nature. For example, Jehovah Jireh means *the changeless One who meets my needs*. Elohim means the God who makes covenants. Jehovah Nissi means *my banner, miracle,* and *victory*. El Shaddai means *the God who is more than enough*. And Jehovah Shalom means *the God of peace*.

When Moses asked God, "What is your name?" in Exodus 3, Moses didn't just want to know how to address God. No, Moses wanted a revelation of God's character, and that's exactly what he received when God answered, "Say to the children of Israel: 'The Lord God of your fathers, the God of Abraham, the God of Isaac, and the God of Jacob, has sent me to you. This is My name forever, and this is My memorial to all generations'" (Exodus 3:15 NKJV).

I love that, don't you? God was saying, "Tell them I'm your God" And He is making the same declaration to us today. No matter what your name means (See Sassy Suggestions) or what grandma name you've chosen, God is saying, "You're my precious child, and I am your God." That seems so personal to me. I love the assurance that we are his and he knows us by name. You are a mighty woman of God and a child of the Most High. Now, go put *that* on a shirt.

prayer:

Father God, I am so grateful that you call me your child. Thank You, Lord, for choosing me and being such a personal father to me. I love you. In Jesus' name. Amen.

sassy suggestions:

» What does your name mean? My name, Michelle, means *Godly woman* or *one who is like God*. I'm sure that wasn't always the case, but I'm thankful my parents gave me that name. My grandson Walter Boone was named after my dad, Walter, and Boone means blessing. So fitting for that sweet little fella. It's actually quite fun to find out the origin of your name or the names of your loved ones.

» If you'd like to look up the meaning of your name, there are many websites that will assist you. Here's one to try: https://babynames.com/name/my

9

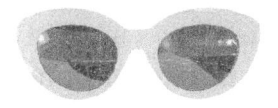

For God did not give us a spirit of timidity, or cowardice or fear, but (He has given us a spirit) of power and of love and of sound judgment and personal discipline (abilities that result in a calm, well-balanced mind and self-control).
(2 Timothy 1:7 AMP).

bugs be gone

Connie Clyburn

I don't like bugs. Never have. As a child, I'd be outside playing when suddenly, as my mother tells the story, I would scream *like somebody was killing me*. She would run outside just to find out there was a bug on the porch step between me and the door to get inside. If a spider gets near me and you're also standing close by, better take cover. That's all I have to say. If you value your life, get out of the way. Getting older has not helped me overcome this fear.

2 Timothy 1:7 tells me God has not given me a spirit of fear. Then where did I get this arachnophobia and bug aversion? Certainly not from God. When I get to heaven, I know I'll be asking, "Why spiders?" No rush, I can wait. Buggy friends who love to study the many legged creatures tell me spiders help to keep the pest problem at bay. All the while, I'm thinking I can certainly entertain a few more gnats just to get rid of the spiders.

It's not just spiders—I'm not a fan of any bugs, really. Any unknown bug flying in my direction has me wildly swatting the air like I'm in a Kung Fu competition. My husband laughs because he can see that it's something harmless, like a moth. I can't hear him tell me that as I flail and run around the yard. I don't want anything flying in my face. You'd think I wouldn't let it bother me so much anymore. I'm a grown adult who should have learned to deal with this by now. My mother smashes bugs and goes on her merry way. Others don't seem to care about bugs. But me … I *spider check* every chair, looking under and around each piece of outdoor furniture before I'll settle into it. My husband knows how I am, so he will often do the checking for me. I guess I don't trust him to look in every nook and cranny, because I do a second look just to be sure.

Those creepy critters can get inside the house, too. I know this because I have had encounters of the yucky kind with those long-legged web weavers that seem to come from nowhere just when you least expect it. I remember well the night it happened. I lay snoozing in bed with my schnauzers snuggled in around me. Suddenly, I feel something run up my back. I came up out of that bed with lightning speed, sending the schnauzers scattering, looking at me like, *what on earth?* Sure enough, a spider had invaded my territory. I shivered, knowing that I would have to take care of the little creature. I grabbed a broom and… kaboom! I overcame my scary spider fears that night and took care of business. I'm glad to report that I'm still developing in that area, as I squashed a small spider crawling across the dash in my car recently.

Oh, my mother loves telling everybody about my bug phobia. She announces it like a ringside emcee at a boxing match. Thanks mom. Now everybody's wondering what's wrong with me. They're probably thinking, *Didn't you raise her right?* It's on you, mom.

The whole bug-phobia thing is on me, I guess. It's my goal every day not to walk in fear—not even with a bug or spider. I can't do it in my own strength. I tried that route and quickly discovered it didn't work. But when I establish my ways on the Word of God, I find strength and ability as I meditate on scripture and declare it out loud over my circumstances. When I declare it, I remind myself that I am an overcomer. It also lets the enemy know I mean business.

I have determined I don't have to live in fear of getting older and what that may or may not bring with it. And I certainly can't let those bugs hinder my future. There's no need to hide out in my house and let life pass by me. No way am I going to let myself be afraid and miss out on all God has for me. He has a purpose for me all the days of my life. I make it my determined purpose to fulfill the plan he has for my life.

prayer:

Dear Jesus, Thank you for making all of creation for me to enjoy. Help me to truly enjoy it. I make your Word my foundation, and I know I am victorious over every fear as I stand. Strengthen me by your precious Holy Spirit that dwells in me. I praise you. In Jesus' name. Amen.

sassy suggestions:

» **Meditate on God's Word.** Find a scripture that defeats fear, add it to your prayers during the day, and meditate on it.

» **Phone a friend.** Find a prayer partner you can call or text to pray for you.

» **Praise.** Put on some worship music and praise away your fears.

» **Count your blessings.** When you thank God for all the great works he has done for you, fears take a hike.

» **Do it afraid.** Take a step toward doing something that seems scary. Ask God to help you overcome your fears, then get ready to walk free.

10

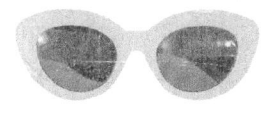

Therefore encourage one another and build one another up, just as you are doing (I Thessalonians 5:11 ESV).

i get by with a little help from my friends

Cynthia A. Lovely

The two elderly women were laughing and giggling like teenagers. To an unknown observer, they probably would wonder what the joke was about or why they were so happy. Perhaps they were celebrating over lunch about a successful shopping trip, or discussing the latest news about a new grandchild. Maybe they were sharing fond memories of former days and busy times of travel and adventure.

None of the above. The two silver-haired ladies, well into their seventies, were talking about the one they loved the most—Jesus. They were believers and followers of Christ, and walking the same narrow path while enjoying true fellowship. These women, my mother and my pastor's wife, were so much fun to watch when they spent time together. I would usually bring my mother to meet up with her friend, so I had many opportunities to observe them. They definitely knew how to encourage and build up one another.

They had many stories to tell from their combined years of living for God. Neither of them ever grew weary of sharing about the goodness of God. Telling story after story of how the Lord had answered their prayers, changed situations, and came along right on time, bringing hope to hopeless problems. The comradery they had between them was precious. Both of them knew the saving power of the blood of Jesus and the cleansing works of being freed from all sin. They had powerful testimonies of the work of God throughout their lives. Through good times and sometimes difficult paths, they stood strong in faith and love of the Lord. Their time together exemplified this scripture of encouragement and support.

These sweet ladies were as busy as anyone else in their separate responsibilities of family and ministry, yet they made time to meet up. Maybe it was the years of wisdom which taught them the value of these friendships. It would be wise to heed their example and check our own maxed out calendars. In today's world of high speed, our souls cry out for the refreshing times of companionship with our sisters in the faith.

I know I have been guilty of putting this off and getting caught up in everyday routines. Through life changes, job transitions, home responsibilities and the latest threat of the pandemic, friend time has sunk low on the list of priorities. Oh, but my heart longs for the fellowship. We are not created to be in isolation. And there is something unique about meeting with a good friend of like faith and trading stories and testimonies, lifting each other up in the Lord.

The good news is age has no limits here. No matter how young or how old we are, we still need each other. As we spend time with our girlfriends, we lift each other up and help to build up our faith together. Whether it is a spontaneous meeting at a tea or coffee shop or a well-planned out day spent with our friend enjoying retail therapy, the time we share is priceless. We can find true comfort discussing problems and solutions, and magnifying the goodness of God throughout our journey. When we talk about Jesus and he is the center of it all, we can leave refreshed, renewed, and edified in Christ.

There is something within us wired for this fellowship and connection in the Lord. If we are going through a difficult time, it may be easy to cancel out, not wanting to add to our friend's own struggles. That is probably the time we need the fellowship more than ever.

Through trials, we can make a special effort to stay in touch. We can connect through phone calls, texts, FaceTime, or zoom calls. And snail mail is also a wonderful option. We all love to get a letter or card in the mail from a friend. When the weather is cooperative, we have more options to gather at outside venues. Picnics, concerts, beach time are all good times together.

Let's try harder to meet up with our friends and celebrate our mutual faith in Christ. It comes with a guarantee to leave encouraged and refreshed.

prayer:

Teach us, Lord, to value our friendships and cherish the beautiful fellowship we find with our sisters in Christ. Let our hearts desire to be one of encouragement and supporting each other. Help us find the time for our friends and to make it a priority. Remind us when we forget, to keep in touch and to nurture our friendships. In Jesus' name. Amen.

sassy suggestions:

» Check your calendar, shift days as needed, and circle a couple of days to spend time with a friend in the coming months. Be open and flexible.

» List possible activities for two or three friends according to their likes and dislikes. One friend may love to shop antique stores while another friend would enjoy visiting a local restaurant. It may be as simple as sitting at the kitchen table over a cup of tea.

» Make plans and touch base with a few other friends with a phone call. Give yourself time so you don't cut the person off too quickly in the conversation.

» Mail out *thinking of you* cards to out-of-town friends with whom you may have lost touch.

» Run through your phone list and send out short texts of scriptures and encouragement while praying for your friends. It will be time well invested.

11

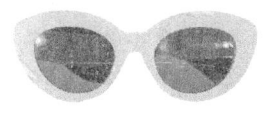

A friend loves at all times (Proverbs 17:17 AMP).

friends forever

Connie Clyburn

I never want to be without good friends. For me, that's a large part of what makes the world go 'round. Be it writer friends, church friends, old chums I've known forever, or cousins who are also my friends, they are all precious to me.

Even though distance and years separate me from many of them, happy memories show up when I see their photo on social media or meet them unexpectedly while out running errands. I've even stalked one or two, thinking I recognized the person standing a few rows over from me in a store as I pretended to be looking at some ugly sweater in the women's fashions section. I want to be sure it's them before I approach them, and it turns out I'm stalking a complete stranger. *Awkward.* Most of us change somewhat over the years, so I guess you can never be completely sure.

The one thing I can be sure about is this—I still love them. Even if we parted on not the best of terms, I still want to throw my arms around their shoulders and give them a big hug. Grudges and hard feelings are just not worth it. People and relationships are worth extending the olive branch. Doesn't matter if I was the one at fault or not, I don't want to stay mad at anyone. And I hope they don't want to stay upset with me. *A friend loves at all times.*

I miss the friends I don't get to see much. The special relationships I've had through the years remain dear to my heart, though distance and time sadly caused us to drift apart. High school friends, college besties, co-workers, and special church friends have left me with lots of dear memories. But I often think of the ones I haven't seen or spoken to in so long and I wonder how they are. Social media has been nice in that respect. It has allowed me to keep up with several old friends and it's nice to know they're doing well.

The years have a way of quickly changing our lives. Marriage, moving away, changing jobs—all good changes, but if you're like me, I tend to get sentimental. I remember the good times and want to go back in time for a few minutes to hear the laughter again and get one more hug from each of them.

Memories of one such friend stand out—the late nights laughing, talking and eating at her house, or the time she spent the night with me when my parents were gone and we thought we heard something go *bump* in the night. A suspicious noise sent us creeping down the small set of stairs in my parents' split-level house, peering around the corner before stepping into the dark kitchen. I grabbed the nearest frying pan as we continued our descent down the steps into the den on the ground floor. We didn't discover the source of the noise, but we giggled about it for days afterward. There was also the time her grandmother told us ghost stories about a haunted house that had me crawling in bed beside my mom when I arrived home that night. Talk about hearing bumps in the night.

I love visiting memory lane from time to time, especially as I see society changing so much. I'm sure the older adults who were in my life years ago thought the same thing and had stories of their own to tell. We all think our generation grew up during the best time.

I include family in my friends list, too. It's so easy to get into disagreements with those with which you're closest. One reason is probably because family members are a lot alike. When Mamaw and Papaw go on to glory, I don't care if I get the matching place settings or not. Relationships with family members are also precious. My cousins were just about the only friends I had growing up. We went to church together, attended family gatherings together, played together nearly every day—too many precious memories for me to throw it all away over a silly squabble. If that's something you're dealing with, I encourage you to take the first step and make amends. It will be so worth the effort, and you'll be glad you did. *Love conquers all.*

prayer:

Dear Lord, Thank you for all the friends in my life. I love each one dearly and treasure the relationships I have with them. You knew I would need friends, and you picked out the perfect ones for me. These special relationships help make life roll along like the tune to a favorite song that comes on just at the right time. I pray a special blessing on each of my friends. I love you, Lord. In Jesus' name. Amen.

sassy suggestions:

» As we get older, it's important to maintain the friend ties that bind hearts together.
» If distance gets in the way of meeting in person, a quick message on social media or a pretty card are great ways to stay in touch.
» Be quick to forgive when misunderstandings arise.
» Celebrate milestones with friends.
» Be willing to help hide the bodies if necessary (just kidding).

12

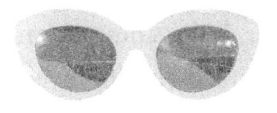

Then you will call, and the LORD will answer; you will cry for help, and he will say: Here am I (Isaiah 58:9 NIV).

superior moments

Cynthia A. Lovely

There may be times in our lives we keep calling out to God, praying, and crying and the answer doesn't seem to appear. We know God promised he would respond. And no matter how we feel or what our emotions are telling us, his Word remains true.

Then … lightbulb moment. We realize, he answered, and he was there all the time. This truth is reassuring to me as I face a time of life where I sometimes have *superior moments*.

We often know them as senior moments, but I prefer my more positive phrase. After all, it has taken me many years to qualify for superior moments. I want to give them the honor they deserve. I had one of these moments on a recent trip to our local library, and the reality of this scripture came alive to me.

My dear husband agreed to stop at the main branch library so I could peruse their new fiction titles and check out their latest DVDs. It was a bitter winter day and he made some statement about waiting in the car. "No, come in and look around. It's way too cold out here." He agreed and followed me inside the building. "Let's not lose each other."

"Oh, I'll find you, no problem," he said. I told him what sections I would be in and started my library search.

As usual, I got lost in library delight, finding new books and a few by my favorite authors. I finally looked at my watch and realized the time had flown. I began my search for my husband. I circled the library with no success. He wasn't in any of the sections I had mentioned to him earlier. I circled again. No sign of dear husband. I checked all the corners and hidden areas. Nothing.

At this point, I was getting tired and cranky. I went out to the parking lot, thinking he had gone to wait in the car. Not there. I looked through the library again, texting him and calling his cell phone only to get his recorded message. I was calling, but he was not answering. Had someone abducted my husband from the speculative fiction section? I left him several messages, becoming more annoyed because he wasn't responding. Walking around again and again thinking we just kept missing each other.

Finally, I found him. Me—annoyed and frustrated. He—calm and serene. "Where were you?" I demanded. He shook his head.

"Right where I told you I would be," he said.

"No way. I looked there over and over again." He took my hand and led me to the magazine section, where he had been sitting in plain view in one of the chairs in the middle. I don't know how I could have missed him. I had gone by that section many times, but my focus must have been on the bookshelves and not the chairs right in front of me.

How many times do we call upon Jesus and he answers us, but we totally miss it? We continue to pray and cry and plead, yet his answer is right in front of us. We become irritated, annoyed, and frustrated. The doubts build up and faith fails. Instead of dwelling on God's promises that he will be there for us, we wander and roam, overlooking the obvious directions in his Word. He calmly waits for us to wake up and see him and slow down enough to hear his voice.

When we call, the Lord *will* answer us. Our eyes and ears need to be open to his response so we don't miss it. On this library excursion, my husband had done everything he had promised. The chaos and confusion came all from my end, not from his. He had been patiently waiting for me to do my part and remember our agreement to meet. This superior moment taught me a lesson on God's faithfulness and my humanity.

prayer:

God, help us slow down, to focus on your promises and not miss the answers you faithfully send our way. You stand sure on all your promises to heed our call and our cry. Thank you for your great faithfulness and understanding when we lose our way.
In Jesus' name. Amen.

sassy suggestions:

» I have had *superior moments* most of my life. I admit as I get older, these moments may occur more frequently. Some people suggest doing crossword puzzles to improve memory function.

» There are other actions which help me to remember in certain situations. For example, turning out all the lights downstairs before I head upstairs. I have learned to say the words out loud. "Okay, lights off," as I flip the switch. There is something about saying the words aloud that helps me remember once I am upstairs. I use the same tactic when I shut off the iron. "Yes, iron off and unplugged." A simple method, but it seems to work. Try it out and see.

» Lists are a wonderful backup plan. Whether a grocery list or to-do list, they serve us well at this time of our lives. Just keep lists in the same place so you remember where the list is when you need it.

» Along with the natural challenges, I hope to be more open to superior moments when the Lord is trying to impart wisdom and direction. "Okay, lights on in my prayer time, shining God's Word in my heart." I speak his Word aloud and remind myself of his great and awesome promises. God can take our *superior moments* and turn them into *spiritual moments*.

13

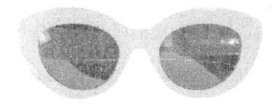

If then you have been raised with Christ, seek the things that are above, where Christ is, seated at the right hand of God. Set your minds on things that are above, not on things that are on earth (Colossians 3:1–2 ESV).

undistracted

Michelle Medlock Adams

When I watch my three-year-old granddaughter, Wren, (or Wrennie Roo, as we like to call her) she wants my undivided attention. Actually, *wants* might not be quite the right word—it's more like she demands it. If I get distracted by a text message or I stop working on a puzzle with her to start lunch, she whines, "Gigi, I want you to *play* with me."

She doesn't just want part of my attention. She wants my complete attention, and I do my best to give it to her. I want her to know that she is more important than texting, cleaning, or literally anything else. I make her a priority when she is at my house, and because of that, she loves to visit.

Guess who else wants (and demands) our attention? Our Father God. Now, that's not to say God whines like a toddler. The Bible says he is a jealous God, but not jealous in an immature and sinful way. He is jealous in that he doesn't want to share our affections. It hurts him when our love for him is diminished by other actions. Wouldn't you be jealous if someone you loved dearly seemed to value jobs, hobbies, or scrolling through social media above you?

He doesn't want us to only *kind of* be there with him. He wants our full attention when we're spending time with him, and he doesn't want us to forget about him when our quiet time with him is over. He wants to be a part of your everyday life, even down to the most mundane tasks.

When we give our whole attention to God, it pleases him, especially in the morning. Giving God the first part of the day lets him know he is your first priority. Don't get distracted with checking Facebook or doing last night's dishes before you've spent time with your heavenly Father.

Distractions are dangerous because they can ruin our relationship with others and with God. In Luke 8, we read about the parable of the sower. The seeds in this story experienced lots of trials that made it impossible for them to grow into healthy plants. Birds ate some seeds. Some fell on rocks and had no soil. But the seeds I want to focus on are the ones that fell among thorns and were eventually choked out by the thorn bushes.

If the seeds represent the Word of God, and we are the soil, what are the thorns?

When Jesus first told this story, his disciples were a bit confused. So, he explained the story to them. "And as for what fell among the thorns, they are those who hear, but as they go on their way they are choked by the cares and riches and pleasures of life, and their fruit does not mature" (Luke 8:14 ESV).

I don't know about you, but those thorns sound a lot like distractions to me. We might hear the Word on Sunday morning and leave church feeling inspired, only to come home and become overwhelmed by all the distractions clamoring for our attention.

What are your thorn bushes? What distractions are keeping you from being fully present with God? And, more importantly, how can you eliminate them?

If I'm being honest, I often have a difficult time being fully present. My to-do list runs through my mind when I'm praying. And sometimes, I let a phone call or a text message steal my morning devotional time. Let's face it—the world we live in is busy and loud, and it's easy to get sucked into the chaos. But it is always so worth it to stop giving into distractions and instead fully focus on God. When I stop and remind myself *what, and who,* is really important, my mind stops racing and peace fills my heart. I've often heard that love is spelled T-I-M-E, and if that's true, shouldn't we make sure our time is spent with God and the people we most value? Go ahead—put down that smartphone, turn off that television and be fully present.

prayer:

Dear Lord, You are most important to me. Please make me aware when my mind wanders, or when I become distracted from you or the people I love. Father, work in my heart to put my priorities in place. In Jesus' name. Amen.

sassy suggestions:

» If you don't already, set a daily time on your schedule for spending time with God. Put away your phone, turn off the TV, and hide yourself away from any other distractions. Even if it starts as a short time, focus on dedicating that time solely to God.

» To practice giving God your undivided, undistracted attention, try meditating. Look at Psalm 119:15 for inspiration. Find a quiet space, clear out your mind, and focus on God. You can choose a scripture verse to say out loud, or you can sing praises to him. Focus on the presence of God. If your mind begins to wander, gently guide it back. Make it a habit to spend several minutes doing nothing but being still before God and meditating on his goodness and his promises.

» Find a Bible reading plan and commit to spending time each day doing nothing but diving into scripture. Keep a highlighter handy, as well as a journal where you can jot down thoughts regarding that passage of scripture.

14

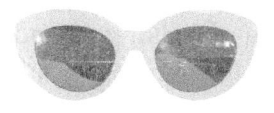

But the one who stands firm to the end will be saved (Matthew 24:13 NIV).

stand strong

Cynthia A. Lovely

Life can get complicated. Distractions come from all sides, and the world around us may feel like it is spinning out of control.

More than ever before, we see the importance of holding on to the truth of the gospel and remaining steadfast in our walk with God. We must endure till the end. Hold on, persist, stand firm.

Yet there can be a slow chipping away at our supposedly rock-solid faith and somewhere along the way of troubles and trials ... we start to slip. The clamor of voices and choices surround us until we veer just a little off the path. We know better. We have so many good years behind us and have been consistent and committed. And we are closer now than ever before to our eternal destination, but we are still vulnerable.

I remember an experience while attending a writer's conference. My husband traveled with me and we enjoyed our time in the Blue Ridge Mountains. There were many hiking trails for him to explore while I attended classes. The retreat was set among the mountains and there was always a lot of walking up and down hills with many levels of stairs in the buildings.

I had injured my ankle before the conference and was leery of tripping or falling, since my balance seemed to be off. My normally klutzy self was in worse condition for a trip, but I was ready. I had prayed many weeks before the event for God's divine protection over myself and also over my husband. On his hiking pursuits, he has come across a rattlesnake and there are black bears in those mountains.

We started the week covered in prayer. I had prayed for protection and for God's angels to guide us for the entire week. Along with the earnest prayers, we both determined to be careful and not take any stupid chances or unnecessary risks. We were prepared with prayers plus wisdom. We were on our guard and I made deliberate attempts to slow my steps, refusing to be hurried. Not always easy at a busy writer's conference. Yet, even though the lunch lines might be long or I could be late for class, I kept to the slower pace.

The extra effort made a difference. We had a lovely time during the conference and on our vacation afterward—still keeping in mind to stay slow and not be rushed. Then it came time to head home. The flight was early in the morning, airport lines were ridiculous, and both of us were tired out by the time we finally got on the plane. It was a safe flight and an easy ride home from our local airport. We arrived home and my husband went into the house first with the baggage. Perhaps I felt safe since we were home and could relax my guard, or maybe I was too foggy from lack of sleep and depleted energy. I followed him in the door and promptly tripped over the threshold and fell flat into my house and onto the living room floor.

Wait, I had arrived home, my safe place. Something was wrong with this picture. I banged up my knee and had a few other aches and pains. My first reaction was confusion, then humiliation. Sprawled out on the floor, moaning about the soon appearing bruises, I felt pretty ridiculous. I couldn't make it through my own front door safely, yet I had managed to make it through 10 days away on an injured ankle without any problems.

Once home, I realized I had completely let down my guard.

I was tired of the journey and not paying much attention to going through my own front door.

I believe God protected us throughout the trip. And I also believe He revealed a truth to me through my personal *trip*. He still answered prayer and honored our attempt to be careful and wise. Looking back, I know I wasn't paying enough attention anymore because I was back on familiar ground.

Time may be closing out in our current world. End time prophecies are coming to pass and every one of us grows older each day. This is not the time to let down our guard. We are called to endure to the end, right until God calls us home. There may be distractions and tricks of the enemy to veer us off course. There is no space left for daydreaming and thinking all is well. More than ever before, let us keep our eyes focused on the goal.

I want to beware of the weariness which may overtake us on this long journey as we get closer to the finish line. We may think we know the path so well that it is okay to relax our convictions and stop paying attention to our steps. Just as I thought I had made it safely home and stopped paying attention, we may be tired and relax a bit too much as we near our goal. Let us persist, stand firm to the end, and we shall be saved.

prayer:

Dear Lord, help us stay focused and pay attention to our steps. As we get older and eternity grows closer, let us determine to stand strong unto the very end. In Jesus' name. Amen.

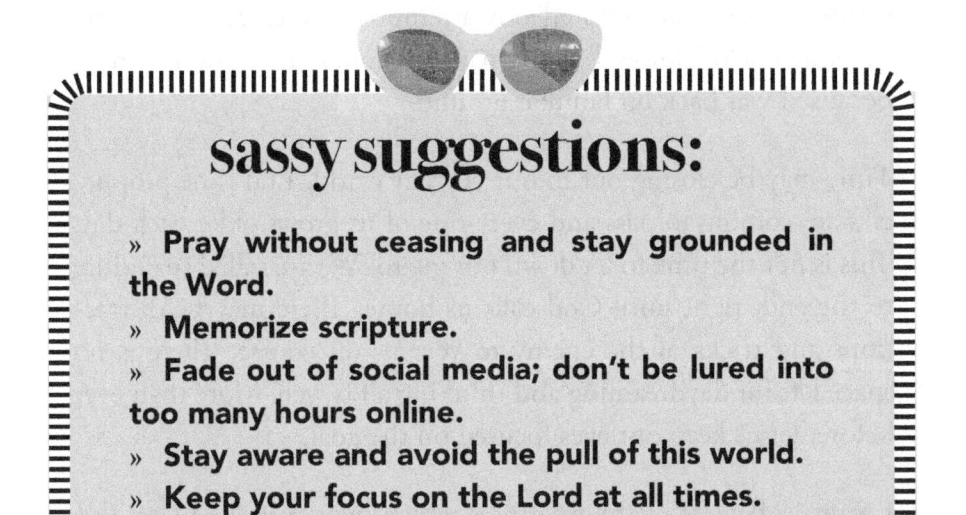

sassy suggestions:

» Pray without ceasing and stay grounded in the Word.
» Memorize scripture.
» Fade out of social media; don't be lured into too many hours online.
» Stay aware and avoid the pull of this world.
» Keep your focus on the Lord at all times.

15

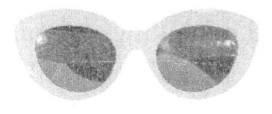

Finally, brothers and sisters, whatever is true, whatever is noble, whatever is right, whatever is pure, whatever is lovely, whatever is admirable—if anything is excellent or praiseworthy—think about such things (Philippians 4:8 NIV).

the golden years

Michelle Medlock Adams

I just had a birthday, and as with all birthdays, I turned a year older. Isn't it so annoying how that always happens?

Amidst all the celebration, I took a moment to reflect on what the past year, and all the years before it, had brought. My heart swelled with gratitude. As I processed just how wonderful of a year it had been, I made a decision. I decided to embrace this senior season and stop fighting it. Although, I'm still going to fight those wrinkles with every fiber in me.

During that moment of reflection, a certain clarity emerged. I realized I have spent my entire life yearning for the life I live now. I finally have the extra time I'd always desired during those child-rearing years and those 9-to-5 hustling and hurrying years. During that season, I spent many days dreaming of a full night's sleep and, if I was really dreaming big, even a bubble bath once in a while.

But now, it's just me and my hubby and our small petting zoo. I'm blessed to be in the financial season in which I work because I love it, not because I need to put food on the table. I have the freedom to pursue my passions with greater tenacity because I have more time and a greater openness to new possibilities. The demands of my 20s, 30s, and even 40s are in the rearview mirror.

Aging doesn't have to mean slowing down and settling in. It certainly doesn't have to look like the older folks in movies who spend their days knitting and doing jigsaw puzzles, unless that's your thing. In fact, for many women, aging means the beginning of a new adventure. (And grandchildren. And eventually, great grandchildren.) In this season, the responsibilities surrounding work and family typically decrease. This leaves more time, and with that time, you have more freedom to choose how you spend it.

Need a quiet space? You can usually get it. Need to pamper yourself? You can usually find a slot in your schedule. Want a night out with your significant other or friends? It's much easier now that you don't need to find a babysitter or worry about the work deadline tomorrow.

But all too often, when we think of aging people, we think of them like Charlie's grandparents in the movie *Willy Wonka and the Chocolate Factory*. It's hard to forget the image of four sad, sickly grandparents all lying in the same bed. Sitting in bed for 20 years doing nothing but complaining and eating cabbage soup. I don't know about you, but I don't want to age like them.

If you've seen the movie, though, you know circumstances change quickly for Charlie's Grandpa Joe. One day, Charlie is the lucky winner of a golden ticket—a ticket for a tour of Willy Wonka's magical chocolate factory. When he tells Grandpa Joe that they'll get to go to the chocolate factory, Grandpa Joe miraculously springs out of bed, singing and dancing. I'm nowhere near Grandpa Joe's age yet, but I'm already realizing just how miraculous that heel-clicking dance was.

It was all because he had something to look forward to—something to be excited about and something to celebrate.

My friend, you've got a golden ticket, and it's worth your best jig. God has adventures planned for you. It's time to get up out of your funk and chase after them.

Take a moment to think about the different seasons of your life. What blessings are you able to enjoy now that you may not have been able to enjoy in other times in your life? What opportunities have opened up for you because of the season you're in right now?

Let's face aging head-on with a positive attitude. Don't dwell on all the negative aspects. Instead, focus on the many benefits of being a senior. There are just as many, if not more, wonderful times to enjoy now. Maybe that's why they call them the golden years.

prayer:

Dear Lord, I thank you for this season of my life. Would you open my eyes to the opportunities available to me at this time? Would you find new ways to work through me? I want to make use of every minute of this life. Thank you for these golden years. In Jesus' name. Amen.

sassy suggestions:

» Look at your calendar. Do you have something to look forward to coming up? Is there something to get you involved in the surrounding community? Something to spark your creativity? If not, schedule something.

» Make a list of items or situations you've wished for throughout your life. They can be big or small. Is there anything on your list that you can finally make happen? How can you get started on those dreams today?

16

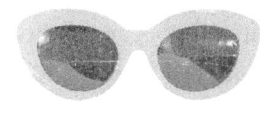

I will never forget your precepts, For by them you have revived me and given me life (Psalm 119:93 AMP).

here's to your health

Connie Clyburn

My recent routine physical remains memorable. Normally, I look forward to it—well, sort of. I don't like needles. Despite that, I anticipate it because my blood labs show if I've been a good girl and added enough fruits and veggies to my diet. It also *squeals* on me if I visited the donut factory drive-thru a few too many times. What about all those apples and brussels sprouts? It's a good thing I like them—give me brussels sprouts any time.

Fast forward a couple of days and my lab results arrive. When the call came, I expected the nurse to say something like, "All your levels are normal .Keep doing what you're doing." The message this time sounded a little different, however.

Wait. Woah. Slow down a minute. What the wha…? My cholesterol is … 206? My blood work has always been near perfect. Then I hear, "Your doctor suggests flaxseed, more exercise, and a better diet." Excuse me, nurse … this must be someone else's lab report. Surely it isn't mine.

Still a little shocked, I frantically began researching natural cholesterol remedies. I went on a mission to quickly nip this little hiccup in the bud. Then I stopped amid my racing heart and my fingers flying across the keyboard. I had let my heart become troubled. I knew I couldn't do this on my own. Right then, I said a prayer for divine help to relax and allow God to lead me. I had to get quiet so I could hear Jesus speak peace to me. I trusted him to lead me in the paths of righteousness—my health is included in that. He would restore my joy and my health as I followed his commandments.

God knows us inside out, so his Word is our best resource. We are unique, with attributes designed especially for us. Who else knows us better than God? He has our cell count down and keeps track of the number of hairs on our head—even the ones that fall out and then get replaced with new ones. *Ummm, Lord, could you make the new ones a color other than gray?* He also knows exactly what we need to achieve the results we want.

Yes, the Lord cares about even that. Instead of scurrying around like a chicken with its head cut off, looking up every naturopath and nutrition expert on the planet, I'll first pray and ask him to lead the way. There's nothing wrong with seeking professional advice or taking medication if necessary. We're blessed with some of the best health professionals in the world.

But I panicked. I let myself get out of sorts. I was mad. My health was out of kilter, and I didn't like it. All my life I've been able to eat, drink sweet tea, and be merry. I like that much better than having to think twice about my food choices. I feel overwhelmed when everything I see in the grocery store is mounds of prepackaged this and frozen that—a lot of junk. There are no good choices. I decide to have air for dinner and call it a day.

I know I'm not 20 anymore. I can't run through a drive-thru with every craving I have for something fried and greasy like I did in college. But sneaking in some fun now and then is okay, too. It seems like a fine line has been set up between our age and food intake. Before age 30, it's ok to *party hearty*. Between 30 and 90, we are supposed to *watch it* and after age 90, it's *no holds barred—you've lived this long, so party big again*. That time in between doesn't have to feel like walking the plank. Instead, dance toward life and joy.

prayer:

Dear Lord, Thank you for relieving all my fears about the future. You have me in the palm of your mighty hand. I will not fear, but trust in you. I can come to you during my panicked thoughts and find rest. You care about my health and well-being. Thank you for always being near me. In Jesus' name. Amen.

sassy suggestions:

» Get some fun paper or a snazzy notepad and make a list of the healthy foods you really like. Then look up recipes using these ingredients and create a variety of ways to prepare the dishes. This way, you keep the creativity and excitement going.

» Love walking, but not necessarily running? Good news—you don't have to run everywhere to get the most from exercise. How about walking or a quick walking sprint? Mark off sections of your normal walking route and do short sprints. Keep it interesting and reap benefits. Always check with your doctor before starting any exercise plan.

» Turn up the music and dance. No need to be a talented dancer for this calorie burner. Dancing is great exercise and it's so much fun. Choreographed or not (work your own moves, girl), dancing around the house will add some fun to your day and you'll get your blood pumping in no time. Now get going.

» Relaxing your mind is also beneficial. Treat yourself to a coffee (or tea) and a good book. Many bookstores offer cozy coffee shops. Next time you're out running errands, take some time to stop, smell the coffee, and read a little.

» Window shopping is underrated. Browsing without buying can provide a downtime diversion after a trying day. It allows the mind to relax and regroup.

17

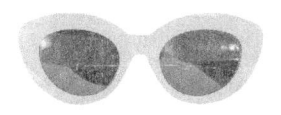

*Open my eyes, that I may see Wondrous things
from Your law
(Psalm 119:18 NKJV).*

i can see clearly now

by Cynthia A. Lovely

It started years ago when my eye doctor mentioned the beginning of a cataract. What? I thought that only happened to old people.

And honestly, it was early for me, and the doctor agreed, which brought me some measure of comfort. It eventually progressed and I knew I would have to address the matter and go for surgery. Vision is so vital to us, and we often don't realize it until it decreases and objects start to blur. It can be unnerving and frightening. Conversations with others who had the procedure convinced me cataract surgery was simple and I would have no problems with it. Perhaps I went into it with too casual of an attitude.

Thinking back on the whole situation, I realized how easily we can relate this problem to our spiritual vision. We want to see clearly, but the world clouds it up and life becomes distorted and blurred. Our view of the Lord and his ways are not as clear as they once were. We waffle on our way and stumble on our path with vision compromised. We bungle our walk upon the straight and narrow.

Yet, the Lord desires to open our eyes so we may see the wondrous. There is an expectation and an excitement in this promise.

In the cataract saga, I ended up with two different experiences. The first surgery was a nightmare. What should have been a simple procedure went haywire and I was sent to a retinal specialist for further tests. The eye doctor seemed concerned with the results, and it took a while for my vision to clear. My eye pressure was up and once he took off the bandage, it felt like a hazy film was over my eye. And the floaters, tormenting specks of black, would float continually over my eye and drive me crazy. The retinal doctor was professional and kind. He kept watch over the eye through several appointments and brought balance to it and hope for the future.

The entire event was overwhelming, and that one eye has never been the same. You can imagine my fear as I wondered if I would lose my sight. As a reader, writer, and musician, it was easy to fall into a terrible thought pattern. So when my *good* eye developed a cataract years later, I put off surgery as long as possible. I was a bit terrified to have another bad experience since there are only two eyes to work with here. However, my new eye doctor kept encouraging me to get it done so I could see clearly again. He was a great doctor, and I had been going to him for several years.

After much prayer and a strong support group behind me, I went in for the second eye procedure. With my supportive husband praying over me in the prep room, I knew God was with me and trusted him to bring me through. I felt his presence, and all the pieces fit together this time. We had a very early appointment, so it was not busy at all. The hospital was a different one and I was familiar with it. The nurses were wonderful and I felt like I was in good hands. This was with my newer ophthalmologist practice and I had faith in this surgeon and prayed for God's wisdom for him throughout the ordeal. Thank God it was nothing like the first surgery and it went smoothly with no complications. I can't explain the burden that lifted from me, having carried this weight too long. Once the bandage was off, I could see—so much better. Each day there was progress. God is good.

Now, I long to see better with my spiritual eyes. My husband and I had gone through many difficult church situations in recent years, and I wondered if my vision had become too blurred and messed up to see God's will clearly. Through this experience, as I prayed for my natural vision, I prayed for spiritual eyes to see once again. I wanted to look upon his face, know his grace, and walk in his ways all of my days.

I prayed to see past the natural realm and into the spiritual world all around us. I asked God for clarity to recognize the schemes of the enemy and to not be fooled by what appears to be impossible to the natural eye. I wanted the Lord to clear away any specks or floaters of distraction, and I trusted him to renew and restore my spiritual vision. I prayed for the Lord to bring back the sweet expectation and joy of seeing wondrous things out of his law.

Every day, I thank God for clearer vision and the ability to see. And every day I pray God will continue to open my spiritual eyes with sharp clarity and focus.

prayer:

Precious Lord, who knows all of our fears and doubts, we praise you for vision—for seeing you as the one and only God who is above all else. Continue to open our eyes daily to view wondrous things from your hand. In Jesus' name. Amen.

sassy suggestions:

» Read your Bible daily and thank God for the ability to read.
» Check your heart on the situations which grab your attention. What do you set before your eyes?
» Research your area for openings to help others with vision problems.
» Ask the local Senior Center if anyone needs someone to read to them.
» Keep your eyes focused on the Lord and his kingdom.

18

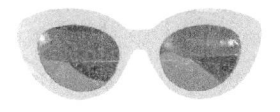

And we all, with unveiled face, continually seeing as in a mirror the glory of the Lord, are progressively being transformed into His image from (one degree of) glory to (even more) glory, which comes from the Lord, (who is) the Spirit (2 Corinthians 3:18 AMP).

mirror reflection

Connie Clyburn

back *away from the mirror.* It was my first thought as I gazed into the small round magnification mirror suctioned to the big mirror in my bathroom. I should have known better. Those tiny little mirrors enlarge your face in a way that makes your reflection look like something staring back at you from a funhouse mirror. And the way it zeroes in on every imperfection. No human being has that kind of x-ray vision, except the people working in the flashy cosmetic store in the mall and my mother.

Since I've gotten … ahem, a little older, it seems like every time I catch a glimpse of myself in the mirror, I get another little surprise. A new wrinkle (fun) or a hair popping out in a place I'm pretty sure the Lord didn't intend to grow there. Wrinkles are lovingly called laugh lines. I may quit laughing. And I don't leave any hairs extending from my chin long enough to give them any love.

I scratch my cheek while gazing in that mocking looking glass and realize my biggest skin issue is dryness. A quick internet search lands on the top potions to help with that particular problem. Good, I'm not getting older—I merely have a bad case of dry skin. Armed with this new information, I race off to the drugstore with the websites saved in my phone so I can buy all the stuff listed in my search.

Once I arrive, I walk in and do a *Watusi* dance with the automatic door, proving that I need help with something other than just dry skin. Inside the store, I go directly to the beauty aisle and find something touted to stop the effects of aging and turn back the hands of time at least 10 years. That sounds good to me. There are only a few jars left, providing evidence it must be a winner since others on the same mission have almost cleaned out the supply. I scoop up the remaining stock and make my way to the checkout, nearly dropping my load of jars and bottles. I never think to get a shopping basket from the stand by the door when I walk in the store.

Back at home, my bathroom becomes a lab as I try each new product and check out the result in that little magnifying mirror.

Try as I might, I realized I can't stop time from marching on. Oh, the creams and products, along with a healthy lifestyle, can help me look my best as I celebrate each birthday, and there's nothing wrong with wanting to get better with age. I've found the greatest anti-aging news is that God himself transforms me daily into the best me I can be. As a child of God, I am continually being transformed from the inside out. I don't know if all my natural imperfections will ever go away, but I can rest knowing God is doing the work in me. When people look at me, they will see his glory shining through. That's a glow I can't get from a bottle or a jar. The only cost is following him.

You may be right there with me doing online searches for the latest and greatest beauty products. Both of us reading the reviews while looking at airbrushed ads of women with smooth skin who claim to be using the same concoction we're considering. It's fun to research and try out new products. I'm the resident guinea pig while conducting my unscientific hair coloring and other beauty experiments. God's way is perfect as he transforms me from the inside out, and I don't have to wait around to see if my hair turns orange.

prayer:

Dear Lord, Your Word says you're working in me to take me from glory to glory. Thank you for doing an amazing work in me that only you can do. I'm excited to follow you on this journey, knowing that no matter my age, I'm getting better as the birthdays go by. Thank you for your perfect love that shows through me to all I meet. I love you. In Jesus' name. Amen.

sassy suggestions:

» **Celebrate big.** Birthday parties are allowed no matter how old you are—go ahead and celebrate each one.

» **Breathe deeply.** Breathe in the fresh outside air. Deep breathing exercises reportedly reduce stress and boost your immune systems. You'll be feeling energized and better about yourself in no time.

» **Laugh.** Laughter is one of the best methods to improve your looks, and it costs nothing.

» **Cat nap.** A short nap anytime you can work it in not only refreshes but allows your body time to regenerate.

» **Water it down.** Remember to drink plenty of water throughout the day to keep your total body hydrated and functioning well.

19

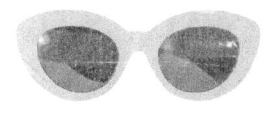

Pleasant words are as an honeycomb, sweet to the soul, and health to the bones (Proverbs 16:24 KJV).

sweet speech & stronger bones

Cynthia A. Lovely

There are a few nicknames my husband uses for me and most of them are cute or somewhat sweet. Cookie Monster (definitely sweet). Kiddo (Aw…) or Snarky-Girl (Hmm …). I'm trying to back away from the cookies and I will always be his Kiddo, but I think I need to work on the snarky title.

I know I should keep the snarkiness in check and direct it more at myself, so no one else suffers from my words. Actually, my hubby says it is more in my writing voice than in my actual conversations. Fortunately, writing can be reviewed, altered, and there is that delightful delete key. However, spoken words cannot be taken back. They drift into the atmosphere and often have long-lasting results.

Scripture teaches about the use of *pleasant words* and reveals the tremendous effect these words can have on others. Sweet to the soul, yes, this phrase is soothing just to repeat it aloud. And who wouldn't want something that would make our bones healthy, especially as they became frailer with the advancing years?

I admit, as we age, we may be more prone to blurting words out without thinking them through. Maybe it is part of the aging process, and we don't have as much of a filter anymore. After all, life is short and perhaps we believe we have reached a point where we can say what we really think or feel. A better idea would be to pause before we respond to some conversations or remarks to be sure our words are sweet. Life-affirming. Kind. Gracious. Words shared that will linger on and lift hearts and souls.

Along the same topic, there is the common and popular practice of using sarcasm with others to garner a laugh. Looking back over some group events, I notice the sarcasm can get out of hand and turn into something damaging. I have been in gatherings of friends where it has almost turned into a contest for who can be the clever one and come up with the smartest comeback during a conversation. At times, this type of bantering may escalate and before you realize it, a sharp remark has hit a target, hurt someone else in the group, and caused embarrassment.

Watching from the sidelines, I have cringed at times. That sharpened barb someone threw at a friend no longer seems amusing. They pretend to shake it off and swing another comment in response, but looking closer, it is obvious their feelings have been hurt. Others join in and before too long, it may feel like word darts flying back and forth across the room. Ouch—duck!

Now, I'm not against friendly teasing. But along with joking around, I try to remain aware of crossing any lines. There need to be boundaries in our conversations and wisdom in our speech. We don't intend to hurt others, yet it may be easy to get caught up in the moment and those damaging remarks slip out.

I love to remember kind words spoken to me. These words have the power to set the tone and shape the frame of an entire day, week, or month. A sincere compliment, an acknowledgement of our value to a project, or something as simple as a *great job* can make all the difference. Yes, these words can be sweet, a comfort to the soul, and a new strength to our lives. We don't want these words to be few and far between, but sprinkled throughout our speech.

There are many ways to offer pleasant words to others in our day-to-day affairs. It may be as simple as wishing someone a great day or thanking the clerk checking us out for her patience with all of our coupons. With our friends and family, we can always share words of hope and healing in this troubled world. Kind words can brighten up our lives and the atmosphere all around us.

Another way to use gracious words is in our writing. I enjoy sending cards to people to cheer their day. A simple note with a scripture can become exactly what someone needs to bring sunshine to their otherwise gloomy day. I send cards to stay in touch with friends, to offer prayers for those who are ill, to thank someone for a kindness they have extended, or to congratulate someone on their latest success. It doesn't take much effort to offer words of hope and support, whether in person, in writing, or over the phone. And our words can bring others that *sweet to the soul* feeling with the added bonus of developing healthy bones. Try it and see. And I'll keep working on my own snarky edge …

prayer:

Lord, teach us to guard our tongues. Fill our mouths with words of hope and encouragement to others. You alone can tame the tongue. Let us speak your words of truth, comfort, healing, peace, and love. In Jesus' name. Amen.

sassy suggestions:

» **Take time to go over your words after a gathering with friends. Would you pass the sweet to the soul test?**
» **Keep your hearts and minds in scripture and let God's Word come easily through your speech.**
» **Write someone a card today with an inspirational message.**
» **Call a friend and express your gratitude for their friendship.**
» **Check out the definition of honeycomb and relate it to this scripture.**

20

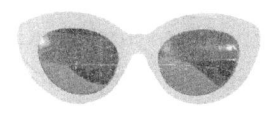

*Give us today our daily bread
(Matthew 6:11 NIV).*

the spiritual senior special

Michelle Medlock Adams

Lately, when Jeff and I go out for dinner, I've noticed as we are walking into the restaurant, *the older folks* are finishing up. I've never really fit in with the early eaters—even though I'm only a year away from qualifying for many of those early bird specials and senior savings. I'm perfectly happy forgoing the senior specials and eating later with the younger dinner crowd. I've always been more of a night owl, so I prefer the evening meal be past 6 p.m. In fact, most nights Jeff and I don't eat until 7 o'clock or later.

But that may change if some of the recent articles I've been reading are correct. As it turns out, there's a reason older folks eat so early—as we age, our body clocks change. By the time we hit 60, we are far more likely to wake up earlier, and therefore be ready to eat earlier, too. There are other reasons as well, such as avoiding nighttime indigestion or acid reflux at bedtime. Maybe you have your own reasons for dining early. And if not, you might just have *that* to look forward to—the joys of getting older, right?

Though our bodies get into a natural rhythm, forcing us to plan our meals, there's a different kind of meal that's not so formulaic.

The Bible often talks about receiving our *daily bread*. In some ways, the phrase is a reference to literal bread. When the Israelites escaped slavery in Egypt and lived in the wilderness, God provided enough manna every morning for each person to eat just enough for that day. Besides being a symbol of God's provision of food, *daily bread* can also refer to God's Word. Your daily bread might be doses of peace, comfort, courage, strength, trust, or faith—all of which are available through God and his Word. Food for your spirit.

Here's the truth about daily bread—it's not served on a schedule three times a day. No, it's only served when we partake of it. To be spiritually fed, we must feed ourselves, and that requires time in his presence and time in his Word. God doesn't just want a 20-minute slot in our schedule. He wants to be intimately involved in every part of our lives, at any given hour. His blessings aren't limited to breakfast, lunch, and dinner.

Daily bread also can't be saved up. We can't get a to-go box of spiritual food to save as leftovers. Just like the Israelites couldn't store up manna for the next day (See Exodus 16), we can't store up our daily bread. We need to partake of God's Word daily. Feeding our spirits only on Sunday mornings—once a week—isn't enough. Week-old spirit food just doesn't satisfy. God wants us to come back continually to his presence and trust him enough to believe he will provide whatever we need, right when we need it.

That hunger you feel for love, peace, and contentment can only be filled by spiritual bread. The same way your stomach might grumble when it's ready to eat, a hungry spirit can grumble, too. And not keeping your spirit fed can be a whole lot worse than not keeping your body fed. Be honest—are you spiritually "hangry" right now? Have you been craving what only God can give?

Spend some time with the Lord today and pray what Jesus taught us to pray two thousand years ago. "Give us this day our daily bread." Thank God for his provision in your life. Read and meditate on scripture to feed your spirit. No matter what time you eat dinner—whether early or late—continually come back to the Lord for your daily bread.

And when it comes to food for your stomach … don't be ashamed to eat an early dinner. Have you looked into senior specials? Some restaurants offer discounts, special menu items, free coffee, or even free desserts—maybe getting that senior special wouldn't be so bad after all.

prayer:

Dear Lord, I come to you to ask for my daily bread. I invite you into every hour of my life, and I invite your sovereignty over it. Help me become more spiritually hungry, Lord, so that I don't neglect you or your Word. Thank you, God, for your provision.
In Jesus' Amen.

sassy suggestions:

» Wear a bracelet, set a cell phone alarm, or leave notes to remind yourself to check in with God throughout your day. Each time you check in, say a prayer, read some scripture, or spend a silent moment in God's presence.

» Before each of your meals, take time to thank God for your food, but also be sure you praise him for his Word—your daily bread.

21

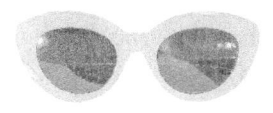

Jesus Christ the same yesterday, and today, and forever (Hebrews 13:8 KJV).

all things subject to change

Cynthia A. Lovely

As we mature, everything keeps changing—our physical appearance, energy level, emotions, moods, habits, and even our bank accounts. Add to that all the changes around us we have no control over—favorite doctors retire, dentists close their practice, friends move away, and our comfortable circle starts to shrink.

I'm finding a few of the physical changes tough to handle. Some tasks I used to do with ease, now feel more difficult. The daily walk (which should be consistent but not always) grows shorter. I used to bike, but right now my balance does not seem to be as good as before. Perhaps, if I *was* more consistent with these activities, I would get better at them—now there's a thought. I tell myself I need more vitamins, which is probably true.

Often, change happens within our own families and we lose loved ones and have to learn how to navigate without them. These changes can create a feeling of vulnerability and helplessness until we remember God never changes. *The Lord, the same yesterday, today, and forever.* What a relief.

The reality of change became more evident to me through an unexpected situation. I needed a dentist appointment, imagining I had chipped a tooth. One of my worst fears—I hate dental work. On calling the office, I discovered my dentist was out for two months with health problems. Panic time. It is difficult to find a good dentist and he was the only one I had trusted. My current dentist was wonderful and had done some intense work for me, which all turned out successful. He was my dental hero. This was the first time he was not available in an emergency. It got me thinking about all the other changes.

My general practitioner had left the practice and they were having a hard time replacing her. It had been difficult not having a family doctor. Then, the lawyer I had planned on returning to for some legal work passed away. My best friend lost her husband and moved back down south. Local churches in our area closed for one reason or another. Our church family no longer existed other than one church many hours away, and life began to feel lonely. Too many changes.

And of course, there were constant and, at times, frightening changes in the world around us. The day-to-day news reports seem to concentrate only on the bad news. Inflation, politics, dissention, riots, crime. Surely there is still something to write about that is good. It is back to the Bible *for the unchanging Good News.* The truth of God's Word remains steadfast and sure. There is One who never changes. God promises to be the same yesterday, today, and forever. Take a deep breath and let those words settle in your heart.

As changes occur daily, we can still look back on all the yesterdays and recall those times God was faithful, over and over again. I remember when I was a young girl, and the Lord drew my mother into a deeper relationship with him. This event caused me to seek God for my own life and to discover the richness of his love. Oh, what a difference he made in my life. Throughout the tough teen years and into adulthood, God led me and directed me. Yesterday and until today, he has been faithful. There is no need to doubt him for the forever part.

I admit I lost it for a bit when the dentist dilemma began. So, I prayed. I prayed the Lord would protect me through whatever was happening. Remember, nothing surprises him. I prayed I would lean into his care and know it was all planned out and he would take care of me, even though I was such a coward and a bit of a drama queen. And guess what? It did all work out—far and above what I expected.

The new dentist was kind and gentle. And surprise ... no problems. Nothing was chipped. I asked her to check the former x-rays and she also checked all my teeth. I wanted to be sure there was no mistake. No issues at all. I flew out of there so fast I'm sure they all had a good laugh afterwards at my escape. This huge to me trial turned out to be nothing. But through it all, I learned to pray about the situation, to realize everything changes *but God*, and because of that, He would *always* take care of me.

I may not be as flexible as I used to be, doctors may retire, dentists may change, friends may move away, and families may shrink. Yet the hope of my life will never change for I have his promise. Jesus Christ, the same yesterday, today, and forever.

prayer:

Lord, we praise you for you never change. Help us always lean into that truth and wrap our hearts around the surety of the One who remains always the same. In Jesus' name. Amen.

sassy suggestions:

- » Make a list of some changes you see in your life.
- » Decide what you have control over and what you cannot change.
- » Make peace with that reality.
- » Embrace change and work it to your good.
- » Help those around you to adapt to changes in their lives.

22

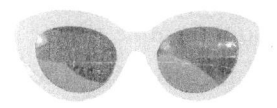

But first and *most importantly seek (aim at, strive after) His Kingdom and His righteousness (His way of doing and being right—the attitude and character of God), and all these things will be given to you also (Matthew 6:33 AMP).*

seeking the kingdom

Connie Clyburn

The day Princess Di and Prince Charles became engaged, I was hooked. I followed their courtship as it played out in front of the cameras, but once that ring went on her finger, she was as good as royalty. The royal family fascinated me and still does.

I often wondered what it would be like to be a royal while watching them attend exquisite balls, meeting with other notables, or just out walking in nature. I could sit for hours reading about the lives of kings, queens, dukes, and duchesses. I loved looking through magazine photos of castles and the goings on behind those stone walls. England seemed so far from my home in the Southeastern US, but my imagination and books took me on many a journey. Medieval stories of princes following a mysterious map to find the king's treasure, and damsels in old stone castles pining away for someone to rescue them from a life of boredom capture my attention every time.

I follow the story and soon realize that each of them is seeking after objects or circumstances to bring them happiness. The main character is depending on something or someone to take them to the magical place of all they ever wanted. They resolve the whole dilemma in a couple hours of sharp acting and movie magic, or in a few chapters of a book where the story ends happily ever after.

In watching the events play out in story form, I realize that I, too, have been seeking after the *fairy tale* that will wrap up my life in a big, beautiful bow of *happily ever after*. If I can just get a book deal or land the ideal writing job, everything else will follow along perfectly and I'll live happily and fulfilled in my little world. Then the thought hits me, *Wait a minute, I'm not a young damsel anymore and I'm still on the journey to finding my treasure.*

Thoughts of panic try to take over as I see myself tumbling off the edge of a castle into the moat below. My fearful mind decides it's too late for me and I get up from my computer.

But God.

The Word whispers to me—*seek me first before all these other things.* I quickly look up the verse, pouring over every word. There's no use by expiration date and no age requirement. There is nothing to disqualify me. I simply need to seek God's kingdom first and he will lead me into *all these things*. There are no limitations and no qualifying characteristics I must meet. My own abilities don't even come into play.

You may be like me—looking at all you've done to achieve your goals. *It's too late,* you might think. Voices in the marketplace shout out that you must be at a certain level at a certain age to achieve results. God says otherwise. His Word simply says, *"Seek My kingdom and My righteousness."*

Hold on to that truth. Put your faith in things that aren't of this world because they won't pass away. Your station in life isn't important. Trust in the One who makes all things new. Follow his plan. It will work for you. As you seek after his righteousness, blessings far better than you ever imagined will open. It's not that you're seeking him to get something—that's not how it works. God has already promised in his Word that if we follow his plan for us as Christians, we will be partakers in the divine rewards that are ours.

You can lift your head with renewed vision. Step back onto the path leading to his kingdom.

prayer:

Dear Lord, Thank you for your precious Word that speaks day and night of the special things you have planned just for me when I follow your lead. I don't have to qualify myself to enjoy the good of your land. Jesus already qualified me, so the results don't depend on my capabilities, my age, or even my station in life. I just follow what the Word tells me to do. Help me every day to focus on you and not the journey itself.
Thank you, Jesus. I love you.
In Jesus' name. Amen.

sassy suggestions:

» Start each day with scripture and prayer. It doesn't have to be formal because you're talking with your best friend—the One who loves you the most.

» Share your dreams and goals with Jesus. He already knows what they are, and he wants to discuss the details with you, offering advice on how to achieve significant results. He is for you and wants you to succeed no matter where you are in life.

» Talk with the Lord throughout your day. When an anxious thought comes, tell him about it. When you get a new idea for a project, seek his wisdom. When you hit a brick wall, talk to him instead of trying to climb it on your own.

» Sing praises to Him. Don't worry about how your voice sounds. You're singing to an audience of one and he thinks you sound great.

» Encourage a friend. Tell them what you've learned by seeking God's kingdom and his righteousness first. Share devotions with them or set up a coffee break to study together.

23

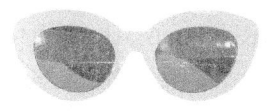

Never doubt God's mighty power to work in you and accomplish all this. He will achieve infinitely more than your greatest request, your most unbelievable dream, and exceed your wildest imagination! (Ephesians 3:20a TPT).

faith at any age

Michelle Medlock Adams

Do you ever feel like you're just not the right age to be useful to God?

This might even be a feeling you've carried all the way from childhood. When you are a child, you're just waiting to hit eighteen. By eighteen, you don't think anyone will listen to you until you are twenty-five. Twenty-five turns to thirty, which turns to forty, which turns to … *I'm getting too old for this now.*

Well, I want to share with you the story of someone who never let age define her or hinder her from following God's call. You may be familiar with Miriam in the Bible. Miriam was a prophetess—in fact, she was the first woman with that title—and she was full of faith from the time she was just a young girl.

When Miriam was around 6 or 7 years old, her brother Moses was 3 months old. The Pharaoh had commanded every Hebrew baby boy to be slaughtered in an attempt to stop the Jewish people from multiplying. Moses' very life went against Egyptian law, and he was getting too old to hide in the house any longer. So, to keep him from being discovered, Miriam's mom built a waterproof basket, placed baby Moses inside, and hid it in the reeds by the bank of the Nile.

But Miriam couldn't just leave him. The Bible tells us she stood some distance away to see what would happen to her baby brother. We can only imagine what she must have been feeling when she heard her baby brother crying and saw Pharaoh's daughter Hatshepsut and her maidens approaching. Miriam could've run away, but she didn't. Instead, she watched in amazement as Hatshepsut looked down at Moses with compassion. And, with great courage, Miriam stepped out of hiding.

"Should I go and find one of the Hebrew women to nurse the baby for you?" she asked.

And, to her surprise, the princess replied, "Yes, do."

So Miriam ran home to her mother, explained what had transpired, and urged her mom to come with her to meet the princess.

"Take this baby and nurse him for me," the princess told the baby's mother. "I will pay you for your help."

Best gig ever. Miriam's mom was being paid to raise and nurse her own son. That's what it means for God to do "infinitely more than your greatest request." I'm sure the whole family was praying for Moses' safety, but God had more to give. Not only did Moses escape death, but because Miriam was brave enough to follow God's call, the family was able to have Moses back in their home for about 3 more years until he was weaned.

But that's not where Miriam's story ends. She didn't do just one incredible assignment in her youth and then run out of callings from God. She grew up to help Moses lead the Israelites out of slavery in Egypt. According to Exodus 7:7, Moses was eighty years old when he first asked Pharaoh to free their people—that would mean Miriam was around 86. Once the Israelites escaped Egypt and started life out in the wilderness, she went on to serve as a leader, worship director, and prophetess. She had plenty of life left in her to serve in whatever ways she could. She lived in service for thirty-eight more years.

What is your calling? If you aren't sure of the answer just yet, that's okay. But hear me out—God has a special purpose, a divine assignment, and a true calling on your life, just like he did for Miriam. You may not have any idea what it is right now, but God isn't trying to keep that information from you. Ask him to show you.

I can look back over my life and see that God was leaving me little clues, showing me I was called to write. I knew in Mrs. True's First Grade Class that I was called to write when I won "Best Poem" in the whole first grade. It was affirmation that I was actually good at something, and I loved it. (I also loved winning glittery stickers and a front-of-the-lunch-line spot on pizza day.) But it wasn't until many years later that I figured out I wasn't just called to write—I was called to write *for Him*. Big difference. It was even later still that he placed a different dream in my heart. I would not just write my own books, but I would publish other authors' books that I believed would further the kingdom.

I could have won that "Best Poem" award, patted myself on the back, and sat back knowing I'd done something pretty cool and left it there. But I didn't. I continued watching and listening, searching for my next assignment from God. I never have let age—young or old—limit how God could use me. And you shouldn't either. If there's one piece of advice Miriam would give you today, I think it would be *He's not finished with you yet*. Never doubt God's mighty power to work in you, because he will exceed your wildest imagination.

prayer:

Dear Lord, Please reveal the calling you have on my life. What do you have for me next? How can you use me in this season of my life? I offer you all that I have and all that I am. In Jesus' Name. Amen.

sassy suggestions:

» Ask yourself—have you ever had an Ephesians 3:20 moment? In what ways has God achieved more than your most unbelievable dreams, and how has he exceeded your wildest imagination? Journal it.

» Look for ways you can serve your church or your community. In what ways could God use you despite—or perhaps because of—your age?

» In your journal, make a list of ways you have served God throughout your life—all the way back to your childhood. Is there anything on that list you might begin again or pursue in a different way? Do you see a pattern?

24

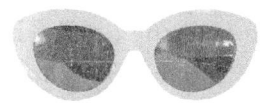

Looking carefully lest anyone fall short of the grace of God; lest any root of bitterness springing up cause trouble, and by this many become defiled...
(Hebrews 12:15 NKJV).

root of bitterness

Cynthia A. Lovely

bitterness. The sound of this word fits well with the definition of it. It comes across as harsh and cold. The Scripture admonishes us here to be careful in case this feeling of bitterness takes root in us. It is sure to cause trouble and problems. Not just to the person who allows this in their heart, but also to others around them.

We certainly don't want to fall short of the grace of God, but if we aren't careful, it can happen. I'm sure we all can remember times when someone has hurt us deeply and we struggle to get past the damage. We know we need to forgive, yet we are human and often fail. That subtle root can lodge within us and cause a spiritual poison to infiltrate our hearts. Because it doesn't always show on the outside, it can remain hidden for years. Under the surface of a church-going, Jesus-loving saint, there may be an ugly root of bitterness growing and developing through time, eventually choking out any hope of healing.

During the years of following the Lord, I have seen many people damaged by this root of bitterness. It breaks my heart. I don't doubt their pain and the piercing hurts they have suffered. I have had my own battles with this issue. But I have also seen what it does to people and I know only Jesus can make the difference and give us the strength to overcome. A few people come to mind, those I have highly respected for a long time. Yet as they age, bitterness that has been in their hearts for years starts to come to the surface.

At the mention of a certain person or situation, anger flares, and cruel words are spoken. Emotions spring to the surface and the tiny root of bitterness from long ago has grown into an untamable beast. It sounds like a horror movie and unfortunately it starts to feel like it. Sometimes these people have been strong and highly favored people among us. We may be so disappointed and disillusioned when we see this come to pass and hear their true feelings. Again, we are all human and prone to fail. Seeing this happen to people I love and respect makes me pray even harder for them and for myself. I am not immune to this problem. None of us are. Yet, viewing what it has done to others helps me to put even more effort into keeping this dangerous root out of my life.

This bitterness not only harms the individual but causes trouble and may defile others. If someone we trust and respect speaks against another person and does damage to their reputation, we will have a choice to make. We cannot condone bitterness and the end results of such conversations. We probably are not in a place to *correct* someone, but we can direct the course of the conversation to another topic. I have done this plenty of times when facing this particular situation. I don't need to debate or discuss what they are saying, but I can turn away from the subject and refuse to add to the growing resentment. It is disturbing to see the results of allowing this root to fester. I hope to be sensitive enough to move past these emotions in others and in myself.

On a positive note, think about those elders who have kept their hearts pure and shine with the goodness of God. I love when I get to spend time with those who have allowed the trials and trauma of life to soften them and mold them into beautiful vessels of the Lord. Their lips speak wisdom. Their faces shine with the gentleness and kindness of God. Hearts still open and pliable in the Master's hand. They may have dealt with hurtful words from people who should have been their strongest support. Yet, they have continually given over the hurt and refused to keep bitterness in their hearts. I recall one Bishop who never speaks ill of anyone. He is one of the kindest and sweetest men I know and has served God all his life. His son once mentioned he thought the church was perfect because his parents never spoke against others. What a wonderful example to their children.

Oh, how I want to age in a good and positive way. May my speech and my actions reflect the changes and molding of God's spirit within me. I hope to give the heavy hurts and wounds from others over to the Lord along the way so he can bring sweet healing. I want to be a seasoned saint rich with the love of Jesus as I grow older. Not a suffocating saint, choking on the huge ball of resentment and poison that has wrapped its nasty tentacles around my heart and spirit. Ouch. Bitterness and resentment—ugly and destructive. Forgiveness—healing and hope in Jesus. I pray as we grow older, we will follow the pattern of faithful elders who allow God to flow through their lives and refuse to keep bitterness in their hearts.

prayer:

Sovereign God, you are over and above all. You alone can heal the hurting heart. Help us run to you with all of our hurts. Lift them from us and dissolve any root of bitterness that tries to grow in us. We desire to be pleasing to you with clean hearts and a right spirit. In Jesus' name. Amen.

sassy suggestions:

» Search your heart. Be honest with yourself.
» If someone comes to mind, bring it before the Lord and ask for his help in releasing any bitterness.
» Pray for them.
» Pray for others who you know struggle with unforgiveness.
» Research scriptures on bitterness, anger, and forgiveness.

25

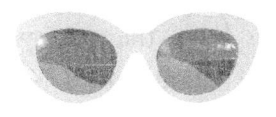

But Jesus Himself would often slip away to the wilderness and pray (in seclusion).
(Luke 5:16 AMP).

a special place of prayer

Connie Clyburn

There are days when I'd like to escape the planet or I'd like to freeze time for a few minutes to stop all the busyness so I could focus on what's important. Sweet quiet time. Just a few minutes with no calls, no other noises, no one asking me to do anything. I don't mind helping when needed, but there are days…

Apparently, Jesus felt that way too (He could have left the planet had he wanted to leave) and he didn't have phones and social media to interrupt him. Just the band of misfits he'd chosen to make into disciples. Can you imagine traveling around with that bunch? I know Jesus was very compassionate with them, just as he is with us. Still, there were moments when he had to get away by himself.

Picture it, Capernaum, AD 27, voices rising above each other.

"I'm the favorite!"

"No, I am!"

"Hey Jesus, we have a question."

I'm sure that sometimes Jesus, the man, wanted to get on a boat and sail off into the sunset alone. I understand. It's not that I don't like people, it's just that sometimes I need uninterrupted time to settle down and spend a moment with my heavenly Father.

It sure would be nice to have a cottage in the woods to go to anytime I need a retreat—a safe, tranquil place to rest in God and *with* him. I imagine a small clapboard siding house surrounded by tall pines. A wide wood plank front porch complete with a swing full of soft, fluffy pillows invites me to sit a spell. Inside the house, a tray of fruit, cheese, and my favorite cookies awaits on a white wooden table. A big pitcher of cold sweet tea sits beside it. Jesus knows this southerner's favorite treats.

While I can't always run away to a cabin in the woods, I can still find a place to spend quiet time with the Lord. In the evening when my husband is watching hunting shows or football games on TV, I can slip off to the bedroom, turn on the fan, and spend quiet time there. At night, when life slows down and it's bedtime for everyone else, I settle into my favorite chair to read the Word and pray. If nothing else, my bathroom can also serve as a *prayer closet*.

A prayer retreat doesn't have to be a certain place. I can meditate on the Word and pray while exercising. On warm, sunny days when I can get outside, walking is my favorite form of exercise (I'm a fair-weather walker). The field in front of my house or the farm next door makes great walking spaces where I can pray while getting in those steps. The surrounding views and barns provide serene scenes as I lose track of time with the symphony of birds as background music. My car makes a great prayer closet. I can sing along to praise music or simply pray in the quiet. It helps me cut down on road rage.

Finding that perfect time and place may seem unattainable, but we can still pray anywhere we are, even in the middle of a busy day. Your place of prayer doesn't need to be fancy or perfect. Whisper a prayer while preparing dinner or sing a song of praise as the biscuits go in the oven. Give thanks for the dishwasher that helps ease the load. At the end of the day, flip off social media and television and switch on a simple prayer of gratitude before falling asleep. It's easy to find the time to pray throughout the day. If Jesus needed to get away alone to pray, then surely we need it as well. He knew the importance of putting aside the busyness of the day to draw from the deep well of communion with God.

Scheduling time to get away with the Lord is one way to make sure it doesn't get lost in the mix of daily activity. It's not necessary to take the whole day off. Even a few minutes at a time will help you refresh and be ready to take on new challenges, like helping your husband find that spool of fishing line he lost.

It's okay if everything doesn't happen according to schedule. God doesn't require a certain amount of time praying. He will not bop you on the head if you don't do everything just right. He *loves* spending time with you and will help you find the time and the place to spend time alone with him. Simply pray and ask for guidance on how to structure your day. Then, listen for the sure answer.

prayer:

Dear Lord, I value my time alone with you. Thank you for helping me make time to spend praying and reading your Word. I want to grow closer to you, Lord. In Jesus' name. Amen.

sassy suggestions:

» **Tea party** - Grab your Bible and a cup of your favorite tea, then head to your room. Shut yourself in for a few minutes as you soak in precious time with our heavenly Father.

» **Just drive.** Turn on praise music in your car and worship while running errands.

» **Walk the walk.** Find a nearby park or walking trail where it's safe to be alone.

» **Alone time.** If you have children at home, send them on an adventure with a sitter, then relish the quiet house to meditate on scripture, worship to praise music, or listen to a devotional podcast.

» **Go to church.** If church is open during the day, slip inside the sanctuary for a mini prayer retreat.

26

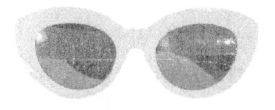

Thou knowest my downsitting and mine uprising, thou understandest my thought afar off (Psalm 139:2 KJV).

sometimes i'm up, sometimes i'm down

Cynthia A. Lovely

Up, down, up down, all the day long. Most of us don't realize how many times during the day we sit, stand, walk, sit, stand, walk and repeat. We simply go about our day fulfilling our tasks as usual, without keeping track of our physical actions. Whether running errands, taking care of our families, getting in and out of the car, cleaning house, or working at our jobs, we are in continual motion of up and down movement.

It is a tremendous relief to realize our great God and Savior knows every time we sit and every time we stand. The Lord's personal and precise attention to his beloved creation is precious. I haven't counted how many times I sit and stand during a single day, but sometimes it feels like non-stop activity. I don't want to even attempt to keep an accurate record of it. And I don't need to because our wonderful Creator sees every action, and he also understands every one of our thoughts.

Many years ago, I worked as a file clerk in a busy state office. I hefted folders, thick and thin, back and forth to file in the appropriate drawers. Talk about up and down. It was constant exercise and a challenge to complete the day's work. The file room took up more than half of the office, with hundreds of tall file cabinets with drawers filled to the brim. Another part of the position involved working as a desk clerk in the reception area. This job required retrieving separate files for other workers who would come in from different departments to request information.

There was even more up and down with this task. We would be seated, take the request, go back in the files, go up and down searching for it, and come back with the correct material. Then we would be seated once again only to shoot right back up for the next request. It could be three or more requests from one person, which could mean carrying heavy, fat folders or a single request slip at a time for one skinny file. Whew. I was much younger back then and able to perform said duties. Now I am a bit older and it would certainly be a challenge to return to this type of job. That was for another time and another decade.

Present day, the downsitting and uprising are still in effect with different expectations and challenges. At this age-not-to-be-named, the downsitting part of this scripture sounds appealing but the uprising—not so much. I'm not to the point of needing one of those fun reclining chairs which practically pop you right back on your feet by the click of a button. I am still able to get up out of the recliner with no assistance—thank you very much. I do admit there are times when getting up from the cozy, laid back couch can be challenging if I sit too long without stretching. There is also the problem of sitting down, forgetting something, like the glass of water I needed, jumping back up to grab it, getting distracted by something else, and sitting back down. Whoops. Totally forgot the glass of water. The up and down starts all over again.

As I go throughout my days determined to *age fabulously*, I remain thankful the God of my youth is the same today and he still continues to notice my up and down life. My reflexes may be a tad slower and my rising comical, but—God knows. He understands my every thought. Think about that for a moment. Every single thought. He not only knows our thoughts, but he also understands them. I can safely say I don't always understand all my thoughts. I can be confusing to myself and my thoughts may feel scrambled. Yet the Lord sees each thought, knows it, and understands it from afar off.

Perhaps the downsitting and uprising also pertain to our emotions. God watches over us when we are down and longs to lift us up again. He knows our different moods and gently guides us to a better place emotionally if we remain focused on him. The Lord also notices when we are up and rejoices with us. We are his children and no matter the circumstance, he will give us joy. The Lord knows our emotional and physical state every single moment. Every time we get up. Every time we sit back down. And all those times in between. What a great and awesome God we serve.

prayer:

Dear Jesus, thank you for watching over us each and every day. You see us when we sit. You notice when we rise. You are conscious of not only our physical actions but also our up and down moods. We are grateful you understand all our thoughts, even when we don't understand them ourselves. You know us like no other. Thank you, Lord. In Jesus' name. Amen.

sassy suggestions:

- » Choose a day and try to record the number of times you sit down and get up.
- » Choose a week and list the up and down of emotions and moods from day to day.
- » Begin an easy stretching routine to become more flexible.
- » Recite scriptures through your exercise, reminding you of all God's faithful promises.
- » Be kind to others who don't move as fast as you want them to. Learn to be patient.

27

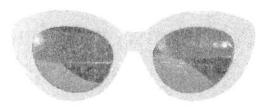

But the path of the just (righteous) is like the light of dawn, that shines brighter and brighter until (it reaches its full strength and glory in) the perfect day (Proverbs 4:18 AMP).

growing up gracefully

Connie Clyburn

The cereal aisle tempts me with its bright boxes promising fun breakfasts with dancing cartoon characters that represent the variety of brands and types of sweet goodness—and a toy. I pause by the Fruit Loops. I want those little rings of fruity goodness. The person next to me reaches up to grab a box of the flakes featuring a little heart on the front, snapping me back to the reality that I'm a grown adult and not a five-year-old. I'm not even a twenty-year-old who can survive on bowls of calorie laden sustenance for days at a time and not gain an ounce of fat nor extra wrinkles from all that refined sugar. I know I should get the bran flakes instead. Bran flakes are no fun. They're … bran. Boring and brown.

Growing up isn't fun when somebody is out there shouting, *"You're no spring chicken! Eat the bran and live longer!"* I don't know who *they* are, but *they* are taking all the fun out of life after you pass the 18-20-year-old mark. If that's not bad enough, the mailbox begins to be stuffed with mail about senior citizen groups, nursing homes, and shuffleboard teams. No offense, but that's not me. I don't want to be included in those groups just yet.

I'm not ready for the recliner. There are goals and dreams I still haven't achieved, and I intend to reach them all, no matter how long it takes me. I might not be a spring chicken by everyone else's standards, but my time clock says I'm right on course to achieve items on my list I'd only daydreamed about while answering emails and sitting in work meetings for years on end. My day job was enjoyable, but the creative ventures I longed for danced in front of me, reminding me to keep walking forward. I envisioned myself as a writer in my home office typing up a storm to meet deadlines.

Vision is important. No matter where we are in life, it's necessary to keep the flame going. My motto is *It's never too late while you're on this side of the daisies.* I try to live by it every day. Oh, sure, there are days when I feel sorry for myself, when it seems like my dreams are underneath the mudslide of other responsibilities that often take precedence. That's when I find myself in God's Word. He sees the possibilities in me. My Father God sees my true future, not the cloud of the enemies' lies that try to pull me down to where I can't see anything but a wall. I know that God's Word is true, and it trumps everything else. It is alive and constantly working in my life.

God is continuously working in us and through us, his children. As we keep walking toward him, our path gets brighter and better with each step. He planned it that way before we ever arrived on planet earth. He designed the way for all who come into the family of believers. We can go forward with that expectation in our hearts because we know God's Word is true and will not return void as we pray and speak it over ourselves. We can be excited about the path we're on, even though it means we're getting a little older.

I've decided, even though my age is increasing with each birthday, it doesn't mean I must give in to what others say I should do or how I should act. In fact, I've adopted a second motto—*Buy the Fruit Loops and don't look back.*

prayer:

Dear Lord, Thank you that my path grows brighter by the day. I can look forward to the future knowing life will get better and better in you. I don't have to stop doing everything I enjoy just because there are more candles on each birthday cake. I will walk in your joy, Lord, and be content in you. In Jesus' name. Amen.

sassy suggestions:

» It's ok to enjoy the fun cereal in moderation. Eat it as an occasional treat for a job well done.
» Keep the vision front and center. Don't give up on achieving your God-given dreams.
» We don't have to live according to others' opinions of what we should, or should not, be doing at different stations in life.
» Find out what God says about you in his Word. His truth is what counts.
» It's OK to have fun in life. Eat the ice cream, buy the motorcycle.

28

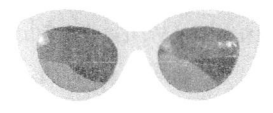

The Lord had said to Abram, "Leave your native country, your relatives, and your father's family, and go to the land that I will show you. I will make you into a great nation. I will bless you and make you famous, and you will be a blessing to others. I will bless those who bless you and curse those who treat you with contempt. All the families on earth will be blessed through you"
(Genesis 12:1-3 NLT).

moving on

Michelle Medlock Adams

Moving is stressful. In fact, according to experts, moving is one of the top 10 stressors in life. (If you've recently moved, you are probably saying, "Amen," right now.) I guess I thought once I reached a certain age, we would be settled and never have to move again. I was wrong. After living in our 14th Street home in Bedford, Indiana, for about 13 years—a home we had completely redone and made our own—we unexpectantly decided to move across town to another home we had previously desired to purchase and redo. It was our dream house. Our Promised Land, so to speak. And so … the packing began.

As excited as we were to move to this home that we'd had our eye on for many years, it did not make the moving process any easier or keep me from being any less worried. Moving is difficult even in the best of circumstances. We were moving in the middle of a pandemic when movers were scarce, and packing supplies were almost impossible to obtain. As I said before, moving is hard.

Just ask Abraham and Sarah. Remember the story? Abraham received a call from God, instructing him to leave his home and head toward a land that God said, "I will show you." Being an obedient and faithful servant, Abraham rallied his family—Sarah, his nephew Lot, and Lot's family—loaded up their livestock and possessions and headed in the direction of Canaan.

Here's the thing, if Sarah was hesitant about moving, the Bible never mentions it. I find that amazing. Sarah willingly went with Abraham without even knowing *where* they were moving. Abraham is the one who spoke to God about this plan, and God simply said it was a land he will show him. It wasn't like Sarah could plug *7777 Promised Land Drive* into her Google maps and have any sense of control in this situation. Talk about a journey of faith.

We aren't privy to the conversation she and Abraham had after God spoke to him, but I believe she said something like, "Yes, husband, I'm with you. I believe you heard from God, so let me go pack all of our belongings and let's hit the road." She gets the supportive wife of the year award, in my opinion.

If I'm being totally transparent, I'm not sure I could have been as supportive. I like to have a plan and a backup plan—just in case. I've been known to have a meltdown or two when facing challenges that leave me feeling vulnerable and out of control. My husband jokingly refers to them as "Missy Meltdowns" (my nickname is Missy). As I've grown up and grown in my walk with God, those Missy Meltdowns come far less frequently, but as I read what

Sarah endured on this journey, I'm positive I would've had at least a few mini-meltdowns. However, if Sarah had any tantrums about the sudden move, the lack of logistics, or her husband's half-truth (saying she was his sister, not his wife, to protect his own hiney—twice!) the Bible doesn't include them. That leads me to believe she remained supportive, positive, and full of faith. She didn't let the physical or mental stress of the move get to her. Sarah didn't meditate on the unknown—she was facing a lot of unknowns in her immediate future. She also didn't get offended at her husband for basically handing her over to the Pharaoh. Rather, she pressed forward, following the leading of her husband, and believing in the plan God had shown Abraham.

That's how we must be if we want to maintain a healthy relationship with our loved ones and enjoy the journey—even when the destination is unknown. I believe the reason moving is such a stressful undertaking is because it leaves us feeling out of control, scattered, and often exhausted. But those feelings can be obliterated if we'll only trust in God and his plan. We can't be moved by our feelings, we must only be moved by our faith.

No matter what you're going through right now, whether you're facing a physical move or some other stressor, the answer is the same. Like Sarah, we need to trust God. Go all in. We don't have to be afraid of the unknown because we serve a God who knows all—the beginning to the end and everything in between. When you know him and you believe he has a good plan for your life, you can embrace life's uncertainties (even moving) with a smile on your face, knowing that your *Promised Land* is just around the corner.

prayer:

Father God, Help me trust you more, no matter the uncertain circumstances. Help me be moved only by faith, not feelings. I believe you love me and have a good plan for me. Thank you, Lord, for helping me trust you as I walk this journey of faith.
In Jesus' name. Amen.

sassy suggestions:

When facing a move, experts agree there are six steps you can take to remain positive.

» **Start with a positive mindset. Don't let your mind dwell on the *what ifs*.**

» **Make time for friends, family, and yourself. Time with your loved ones will lighten the mood and keep you balanced. Self-care is important.**

» **Give yourself plenty of prep time by allowing for missed deadlines and unforeseen obstacles.**

» **Connect with fond memories. Don't be afraid to remember great moments shared in the house you're leaving behind.**

» **Picture your new home. Think about the new memories you'll be creating in the new space.**

» **Ask for help. You'll need help, so ask.**

29

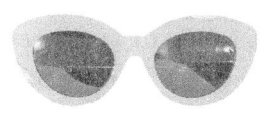

It is better to live in a corner of the housetop than in a house shared with a quarrelsome wife (Proverbs 21:9 ESV).

don't be a qsw

Cynthia A. Lovely

The man leans a tall ladder against the side of the house, adjusts his backpack, and begins to climb. He reaches the top and takes careful steps onto the roof while the irritating drone of his wife's voice fades into the distance. He pulls a small cushion from his pack, settling himself on a flat corner of the roof. With a sigh of relief, he takes out his iPad and earbuds to escape to his own little world, away from any quarrels.

Back in the days of the Bible, this probably looked different and I imagine the roofs were flatter and more accessible. But I can't help it; this scripture brings this comical image to mind. No matter the argument, I doubt we want to drive our husbands out the door, climbing up the rooftop to get away from us.

Looking more carefully at this verse, it states, "To live in a corner…" Ouch. Not just a temporary break, but a definitive exit from normalcy and to actually *live* in this new escape. Let's take a look at the quarrelsome wife. She sounds like a stubborn, relentless woman who has serious issues in communication. We probably don't know the whole story so there may be deep wounds from her past causing her to react this way and always be quarrelsome. Regardless, I know I don't want to be this type of wife and I'm sure you don't either.

I admit marriage takes work. Along with commitment, trust, patience, forgiveness, love and all those other good words we think of for happily ever after. Yet we live in a troubled world and there will be times when the stress and cares of this life become too heavy. Add to that the physical and emotional changes women face as we grow older and tempers can flare more easily. Oh yeah, and once you're both retired, it may feel like you're bumping into each other every time you turn around. Surely the house has shrunk. Maybe you feel like there is no private space anymore. This could lead to sharp words spoken and you may end up wishing your beloved out on that rooftop for a while. However, I doubt any of us want to be labeled as a quarrelsome wife and be the cause of a hubby roof-dweller.

There is a popular saying about choosing your battles carefully. We can pray for wisdom and ask God to guard our tongues in the heat of a disagreement and be willing to step away and give one another space to cool down. I am fortunate to have a spouse who is fairly even-tempered, so we don't argue often. Of course, situations do come up and a disagreement will arise. This is sure to be present in any marriage, no matter how perfect it may look to outsiders. However, we have found a few methods that have helped our marriage.

We know you're not supposed to end the day angry with each other and go to sleep holding a grudge. So during difficult times, we tuck in for the night, barely speaking with an uneasy truce between us. The problem is not solved, but we usually know when to quit if we're both exhausted and capable of saying words we'll regret. We turn out the lights and all grows quiet. In the darkness and the stillness, one of us will eventually crack and break the silence with a defiant, "I love you anyway." The appropriate response from the other spouse is a sarcastic, "I love you in spite of."

Okay, we may not be truly sincere, but saying those words out loud brings the meaning to life. It usually strikes the right chord and breaks up the tension with both of us laughing at each other. Now if this method fails, try our next one—a pillow fight. You just can't remain mad at someone during a pillow fight. Plus, no matter how hard you hit each other, usually no one gets hurt. Just don't use heavy weighted pillows.

I hope these methods are helpful for the next time a situation gets hot and heavy and you're trying to be wise with your words. Let's save our husbands from becoming roof-dwellers.

prayer:

O Lord, help us guard the words of our mouth. Especially in stressful times. Please guide us with your peace and deliver us from quarrels. In Jesus' name. Amen.

sassy suggestions:

» Advancing age and retirement brings change. If your marriage feels strained, perhaps you both need a get-away. All of us have had added stress in our lives with the restrictions, isolation, outside pressures and fears of the unknown with the pandemic. It is time to be creative and take a day away together.

» Visit a small village nearby and walk through their downtown area. Find a park with hiking trails or a place to have a simple picnic. There are many inexpensive actions couples can take to strengthen their marriage.

» We have been to a few church couple retreats. They were a combination of scriptural teaching, beautiful worship, and fun fellowship with other couples. Keep watch for this type of opportunity.

» Of course, a getaway together is good but also be open to personal time. Maybe the wife needs a girlfriend day, or the hubby needs some hanging out with the guys time.

» Know how and when to discuss topics. And most important of all, learn how to *listen* to each other. These are the golden years, but we have to put effort into them to make sure they shine like gold.

30

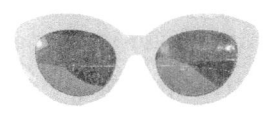

How fair and beautiful you are, my darling. How very beautiful! Your eyes behind your veil are like those of a dove; your hair is like (the shimmering black fleece) of a flock of (Arabian) goats that have descended from Mount Gilead
(Song of Solomon 4:1 AMP).

the poetry of marriage

Connie Clyburn

I smiled as I got into my car at the end of the workday to find a card with a handwritten poem and a stuffed bear. No, some weirdo had not gained access to my car in the middle of the day. It was a poem written just for me by my boyfriend (who later became my husband). He had tricked me into giving him my keys and left the gifts for me. We first met when I went to work for the local sheriff's department. He had been working there for a few years before I showed up. The poetry must have worked its charms, because 30-plus years later, we're still together.

Over the years, the poetry ceased to show up in my car as we settled into life together. Oh, we still loved and cherished each other as we had promised while reciting our vows in front of family and friends. Carefully crafted poetic verses gave way to other favorite activities like Sunday visits to the bookstore and late-night Shoney's runs after he got home from a 3-11 shift as a deputy patrolling our county's back roads. Beach trips and shopping also became our faves. Lots of shopping. Instead of gazing into each other's eyes while reciting mushy poems over zinfandel, we ran the roads and doted on our pets.

What happened to my poems? It was fun and special to find those little notes penned just for me. It seems they disappeared into the routine after the "I do's" were sealed with a kiss. *Had his devotion waned?* Even King Solomon had time to write lines of love to his beloved while running an entire country. I must admit, I'm not sure how I would have responded had my husband commented that my hair reminded him of a goat's hair. We raised goats at one time. I don't ever remember their hair being something I wanted compared to mine.

Of course, he still loved me. I had to dismiss those crazy thoughts that came at me like darts. In fact, the goat story proved his undying devotion. I'm the one who had dreams of becoming a goat farmer. A couple of friends once gave us two female goats to roam around our nearly four-acre mini farm. My husband went to work reading all about raising goats. He bought their food, gave them goat vitamins to keep them healthy, and nursed one back to health after a dog attack. I look fondly back on that time. He didn't start writing me poetry again, but he did look after my animals. That says a lot.

The poetry bug found its way to me, however. Sitting at my desk or the kitchen table surrounded by all my writing wares, I get lost in creative thought as I try to write just the right verses for my husband's birthdays and our anniversaries. I'm terrible at remembering to buy cards and there have been occasions when I didn't have a card for him. Cards are his *love language*, so I knew I had to remedy that. Now my desk drawers are full of cardstock, envelopes, and ink stamps, as well as a cheap fishing tackle box which I turned into a craft box toting colored pens, highlighters, stickers, and the like. I have found new enjoyment in giving him cards. He never knows what crazy rhymes are next.

It's fun to find new ways to surprise him. We always buy ourselves the items that could turn up as gifts at birthdays and Christmas, so it's been challenging to find ways to surprise him. I try to keep my ears open when he talks about spices and utensils he wants for smoking meat, or catch a hint about his favorite hunting brand. I go shopping armed with any clues I can get him to spill without revealing my intentions. The effort put into keeping the *mushy* in a marriage makes for some interesting and hilarious milestones along the way.

Even if you're not the creative kind, there are ways to keep the *fun* in forever. All it takes is a little imagination and time. They will appreciate even the smallest gesture. Perhaps it will also inspire your husband to think outside the tried and true and create little surprises for you, too. He may not know how to write verses to describe your dove-like eyes like Solomon did, but he will find a way to show how much he thinks of you.

prayer:

Dear Lord, Thank you for providing examples in your word to guide us into happy, fulfilled, and fun marriages. In Jesus' name. Amen.

sassy suggestions:

» Keep your marriage ties strong by reading devotions together. Pick out scriptures on your own or find a devotional to use as a guide.

» Remember those early days of dating? A dinner and movie date is still a winner—you can even sing to the oldies together in the car.

» Go to a concert. A lot of the old bands are still touring, and a night out is still the ticket to keep the marriage magical or revive a flickering flame.

» Try your hand at writing a verse or two to your spouse. Pull out the *Song of Solomon* and let it inspire you. Encourage your husband to do the same—you might be pleasantly surprised.

» Hold hands. The soft touch of his hand in yours even after years of marriage will be as special as the first time he took your hand.

31

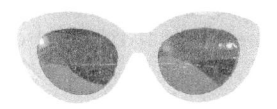

Wherefore, my beloved brethren, let every man be swift to hear, slow to speak, slow to wrath (James 1:19 KJV).

sunset and strife

Cynthia A. Lovely

It was a glorious day for a cruise around Long Island Sound. We were eager to join our friends from our favorite Long Island congregation and be part of this couples group event.

We had the best intentions and certainly were not thinking about any scriptures regarding anger. No anger here. We were set to have a marvelous time. Besides, we knew the value of listening, being careful of our words, and avoiding silly squabbles. With high hopes for the evening, we met up with other lovey-dovey couples intent on enjoying the sunset cruise.

We sailed along smoothly and caught up with our friends we hadn't seen in a while. I had remembered to take a motion sickness pill, so I felt I was handling the waves and rocking motion pretty well. They served us a delicious meal and we continued to float along, admiring the views. The Lord provided a beautiful sunset as a backdrop to our romantic time together.

After the cruise, we got in our car to head out.

Before the event, we had driven almost four hours in heavy traffic, been in a long church service, and driven even further for the cruise. So, we were both tired by this time. Though we knew our way around the island, this activity was not in a location with which we were familiar. No worries usually, but this was without GPS and we had spotty cell service to call anyone for help.

My husband is usually good with directions and finding his way around unfamiliar territory. But at this point, it was getting dark and right out of the boatyard it felt like we were headed in the wrong direction. "Honey, are you sure you know the way back east? Nothing here looks familiar," I asked.

"We'll be fine," he said. We drove along for a bit and I could tell he wasn't as sure as he pretended to be.

"Why does that sign say NYC? We don't want to go anywhere near the city," I said. I felt a bit of panic. I hated NYC traffic.

He frowned and continued to drive along the dark, lonely highway. If you have ever been to Long Island, there are parts where it feels like you dropped off the edge of the earth. And it is true to its name—Long. There are areas where the highway seems to go on forever, especially at night when your vision is restricted. No houses, no lights, no people, and maybe an occasional road sign.

My determined husband turned around a few times and tried to backtrack. It felt like we were going in circles. We were both getting cranky. And then he mentioned we should have gotten some gas. "What? We're out in the middle of nowhere and we're going to run out of gas? Why didn't you think of that before? We're really lost, aren't we?" I was no help. It was pitch black and desolate except for sand dunes and vast amounts of ocean around us. It felt like a sea monster would cross the highway at any moment.

So after our lovely, relaxing, romantic sunset cruise, we were struggling to find our way back and throwing words back and forth a little too quick and a little too harsh. There wasn't a lot of swift to hear, definitely not slow to speak or slow to wrath. We both knew better, but the weariness and travel fatigue plus the feeling of helplessness were a bit too much. And of course, there were no gas stations to be found because we were at the end of civilization.

Oh my, this was not the way to end our evening. Looking back, we can now laugh about it. Our sweet couples event ended up in a spit and spat conflict on the way back to where we were staying.

Once we finally found our way and the correct direction onward, we both began to calm down. We hadn't been swift to hear each other's concerns. Or slow to speak out of our frustration, fear and fatigue. And the wrath part kicked in too quick with all the above emotions playing havoc.

On a good note, we had been married long enough to recognize our mistakes and be willing to talk it through. We had gained some wisdom through the years. We both apologized and eventually had a good laugh about it.

By the time we reached our destination, it felt like we needed another getaway from our getaway. Maybe a Marriage Matters seminar was in our future with clear directions mapped out beforehand.

prayer:

Lord, help us be willing to listen before we speak and to take time to think before we say words we cannot take back. Life will always bring ups and downs, so teach us how to navigate those difficult times without resorting to anger. In Jesus' name. Amen.

sassy suggestions:

» When you feel those emotions rising up in situations, take a deep breath.
» Take another breath and resist the temptation to say words you may regret.
» Try to say a quick prayer for wisdom.
» Focus on not blaming others when a conversation becomes full of conflict.
» Bring the discussion back around by trying to help find a reasonable solution.

32

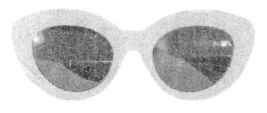

Who satisfies your years with good things, so that your youth is renewed like the (soaring) eagle. (Psalm 103:5 AMP).

kid stuff 101

Connie Clyburn

One beautiful sunny day, I challenged my husband to be a kid again. I grabbed his hand and away we went to the pasture just beyond our backyard. He first looked at me like I'd lost my marbles, but somehow, I talked him into it. Soon we were lying in the tall swaying grass, gazing up into the blue sky, watching the fluffy clouds go by. Good thing our neighbors weren't home at the time.

My ideas are usually anything but boring. My weird ideas are often so I can get pictures for my social media posts, or to use as fodder for my next blog. I also thought we could have fun remembering days from our childhood when we rolled down grassy slopes, ate sour grass, and played games of Red Rover. I wanted to add a little adventure to the day and renew our sense of youth. Having fun will do that—even if it seems a little offbeat.

Harebrained schemes aside, I'll reminisce about fun I had as a child and decide to try reliving some of it. One not-so-fun event of my youth happened the day I ran along the top of an embankment in front of my papaw's (grandfather in the Appalachian South is spelled p-a-p-a-w) big white two-story house trying to catch up to my cousins who were ahead of me. At some point, I lost my footing, slid on the slick grass, and almost fell to the road below. I grabbed onto something like a root or a shaft of grass to pull myself back up. Whew! Another example of the younger me trying something before fully thinking it through involved diving into a swimming pool. Everyone else did it. Why not me? I forgot everyone except me could swim. I flailed around like a catfish caught on a hook, sending water down my nose as I gulped a mouth full. It probably wasn't as bad as I imagined it to be, but still. Some of my youthful adventures were fun and a few ended up being treacherous.

It's no wonder God wants us to approach him as little children. He wants to satisfy our mouths with good, so that our youth is renewed like the eagles. It means trusting him fully. It could also mean lying in tall grass, smelling the earth, and breathing in the fresh air, along with a gnat or two. Kids enjoy the sights, sounds, and smells of creation all around them. The adult me can become jaded. I stare out the front window complaining about the heavy rain pouring from clouded skies, or I fuss about the crispy grass crunching under my feet when it doesn't rain enough. The much younger me would walk outside in the cool rain. Droplets of water rolling down my forehead, dripping off my chin, straight from the clouds way up overhead. That's a long way to fall. Yet, the rain feels soft on my face. I like to go outside after a rain and breathe in the fresh scent of pine in our yard. The rain enhances the many natural fragrances found around my yard. God uses his glorious creation to renew my youth.

I want to learn to live with abandon like a child. I long to let go of apprehension and take off running through a field of wildflowers and daisies sometime. Throwing caution to the wind, I won't worry about what people think. In fact, I'll own it even if I look a little whacky. Kids allow themselves to be who God created them to be. In fact, they don't know how to be anything else. They're clear about their likes and dislikes. Try feeding a kid something he or she doesn't like. I remember sitting at the kitchen table staring at a plate of hominy set before me, that I was determined I would not eat. Was it my fault I thought the bowl in front of me contained corn? One bite told me it was … *yick*… hominy. I didn't and still don't like it one bit. God uses taste and smell to renew my youth even now.

I'm sure God won't make you eat hominy if you don't want to, but he is asking you to trust him without limits. Let him fill your mouth with goodness and renew your passion for life. Give him all those adult worries. He's the same God you trusted as a child. He wants to take care of your grown-up worries just like he diffused your childhood fears all those years ago. He will use his peace to renew your youth.

prayer:

Dear Lord, Thank you for being near me now as you were in my childhood. Forgive me for letting worries distract me from laying everything at your feet. Thank you for loving me the same throughout my life. I commit now to trusting you with everything I face. Help me grow in this area. Thank you.
In Jesus' name. Amen.

sassy suggestions:

» Laugh. Watch a funny movie with friends and giggle the night away.
» Grab a couple of friends, set up an ice cream sundae bar, complete with sprinkles and chocolate sauce, then see who can make the best sundae.
» Dance to your favorite *muzak* tunes in the grocery store. I dare you.
» Get a coloring book, some vibrantly colored crayons, and have fun. No need to spend a lot of money, the nearest dollar store will have everything you need.
» Snuggle up under your favorite warm, fuzzy blanket with your Bible and sit in God's lap for a while.

33

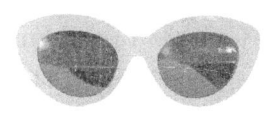

I have not stopped giving thanks for you, remembering you in my prayers
(Ephesians 1:16 NIV).

memory lane of thanks

Cynthia A. Lovely

There are people in our everyday life who are special and loved but who we take for granted. Caught up in daily routines, life rolls along and we may lose the ability to treasure and cherish one another. And we may also forget to keep them in our prayers.

This became more obvious to me when my husband and I celebrated our 35th wedding anniversary. I started thinking about our life together and all the ways I was thankful for my husband. As I listed many memories, my thanks increased and so did my prayers for him.

My sweet spouse has always been a giving person who loves to make others happy. When we were first dating, he would surprise me with simple gestures of kindness. He found out one winter we hadn't bothered setting up a Christmas tree in years. On Christmas Eve, he showed up with a fresh, scented tree at my home. He had raided a closed holiday lot, grabbed a tree, and left a note with money to pay for it.

We set it up that night. Honestly, I think my mother loved it more than any of us. She had missed the pretty lights and holiday atmosphere. I was grateful for this thoughtful gesture. I gave thanks to the Lord and continued to pray for this man who needed to find the Savior for himself.

Then there was the time he bought me a new bicycle. He brought the shiny red bike to my office one day. It was another unexpected gift. I invited him to our church Christmas program, where he encountered the presence of God and began his Christian walk. I gave thanks for this Christmas miracle and continued to pray for him.

God brought us together in his perfect timing and the journey has been amazing. My husband still brings me flowers and chocolates (always a win) and continues to grow in his walk with God. Now we are growing older together and it is a different scenario of items and events for which I'm thankful.

When my elderly parents needed more support, he was there by my side, helping in any and all ways with their care. I remember when my mother died just before the holidays. I was dreading Christmas and all the memories. Yet Dwayne outdid himself by giving me a beautiful blue leather-bound book, inscribed in gold lettering, "Writings of Cynthia A. Lovely" along with a leather briefcase to encourage me in my writing endeavors. I cried and wrote a dedication to my mother inside the cover of the book.

One of his latest attempts to support me is dear to my heart. We live in the country, five miles up a winding road. Our winters are rough in upstate New York with snow and ice. Our front porch can get slick from snow and melting ice falling from the roof. Sometimes when I walk out the front door, it feels like I'm about to slide right across and topple down three steps onto the brick walkway.

I had mentioned to him a few times how I needed a porch railing. Nothing fancy, just a rail by the stair portion so I had something to hold on to. Though he has been so busy at his job, he found time to install a simple wood railing. Three pieces of wood that meant everything to me.

Now when I go out the door, no matter the weather, I grab hold of my railing and thank God for my husband. Flowers, candy, and gifts are lovely, but this type of gesture speaks volumes to me. And every time I go down those steps, I give thanks and pray a blessing on this dear man for his thoughtfulness and care.

Who are you thankful for today? It may be a husband, your son or daughter, your parents, a sibling, or perhaps a close friend. It is a blessing to go down memory lane and recall certain people in our lives we are grateful for and to be reminded to keep praying for them. Let's treasure and cherish these relationships and vow to keep family and friends in continued prayer.

prayer:

God, help us be thankful for the special people in our lives and not to take them for granted. Teach us to remember them daily in our prayers, along with our thanks for all those who are dear to us.
In Jesus' name. Amen.

sassy suggestions:

» Make a list of the people in your life you have been most thankful for through the years and use this as a daily prayer guide.

» For your husband or one of your children, think of a simple way to express your thanks for all they mean to you. It could be as easy as making them their favorite dinner or spending quality time with them.

» Perhaps it is a close friend. Most people would appreciate an invitation to lunch or maybe meet up at a local tea room. If they have a busy schedule, do all you can to make it convenient for them and their availability.

» It may be a friend or relative who has moved far away, so you have lost touch with them. Mail out a card. Or make the effort to place a phone call to catch up on the news.

» Be creative in ways you can express your thanks. Some people like gifts. It doesn't have to be expensive. A small, thoughtful gift can mean a lot.

34

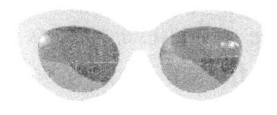

I would have despaired had I not believed that I would see the goodness of the LORD in the land of the living (Psalm 27:13 AMP).

surprise! when life delivers the unexpected

Connie Clyburn

I didn't wake up that day expecting to see an ostrich in my backyard. Early one morning, several years ago, when my husband and I moved into our new house outside of town, I took my miniature schnauzer, Barney, outside for his morning constitutional. A nip in the air meant we wouldn't be out there very long. Barney didn't need a leash, so he meandered around the yard, sniffing every tree while I followed close behind with a flashlight. Dark out in the country with no lights around is the kind of dark you can reach out and touch. On the flip side, the night sky away from the glow of streetlights and flashing business marquees provides a panoramic view of the stars and planets.

My husband sometimes worked the night shift as a sheriff's deputy. He came home after I'd gone back in with Barney and asked if I saw the ostrich out in the yard. My answer—*I was just out there and saw no ostrich. You, on the other hand, have worked all night*. It took some convincing for me to believe he was not seeing things. That and him shining the lights of the cruiser down the tractor path leading to the barn at the back of the pasture. Sure enough, there stood an ostrich. Apparently, it made its rounds to other houses. Later that morning, the ostrich reportedly spied in the kitchen window of my 90-year-old neighbor's house. She was none too happy about that.

I love that kind of unscripted happening. You can't make up stories about situations that happen out in the country. Give me fun unexpected occurrences and I'm a happy camper. Someone somewhere said, "Expect the unexpected." I like to think this is talking about good. I admit I get into the mode where I think something unexpected is always going to be bad. A phone call in the night as I sleepily fumble for the phone means something bad has happened. Somebody mouths the words *"I need to talk to you"* in my direction and I'm wondering what I've done. I always start that conversation by asking, "What have I done wrong?"

What if I turned my expectations around and looked for good to happen? Consider the woman in the Bible who was dragged out into the town square after being caught in adultery. She expected to be humiliated and maybe even stoned. The Pharisees wanted to condemn her. Jesus did the unexpected. Instead of calling her out, He extended mercy. Jesus showed her goodness.

Just like that woman, we receive God's best. We can always count on good from our heavenly Father. As we put his kingdom first, we can expect the goodness of the Lord to meet us at every turn. It's easy to think the *unexpected* means something terrible is going to happen. But with God, it's just the opposite. He longs to give us good things. He wants to surprise us with gifts. I'm going to change my way of thinking around and expect God to add *all these things* as I live in his presence, putting righteousness first.

The Bible is full of promises that God's children can expect his goodness. Psalm 23:6 also assures that he wants us to have the best—*goodness and mercy and unfailing love will follow us throughout our lives.* How magnificent to know the Lord is following us and literally chasing us down with his wonderful, amazing love. He is faithful to his promises concerning us. That's good we can expect time after time.

I plan to change my expectations. No more expecting every phone call in the wee hours is an unwelcome announcement. No more thinking every noise my car makes is going to end up costing me thousands. That headache, the enemy tries to tell me is something serious, is no more than just a simple headache. The devil loves to get us thinking *what if* as he paints pictures of the worst scenarios. He doesn't get to control my life or my future. God's Word is the final authority and I know that means God intends the best for me. I will take those worrisome thoughts to the Lord and leave them there.

prayer:

Dear Lord, Thank you for taking the burden of worry from me. You never intended for me to carry such a heavy load. Thank you for the assurance that you want only the best for me. I can expect good things from you every day. I will rest in knowing that your goodness is chasing me down, bringing your best to me.

I make it my aim to put your kingdom and your righteousness first, and I can expect good things to be added. Thank you, Lord. In Jesus' name. Amen.

sassy suggestions:

» Wake up each day expecting good things to happen.
» Encourage a friend to join you in changing those expectations to looking forward to something.
» Ask God to help you and expect that he will.
» Learn from God's Word how to seek after his kingdom and his righteousness.
» Expect that the unexpected will be something good.

35

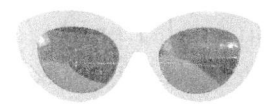

He will yet fill your mouth with laughter and your lips with shouts of joy (Job 8:21 NIV).

life is better with laughter

Cynthia A. Lovely

There are times in our lives when we need a good laugh.

Circumstances may not look bright, and laughter may be the furthest thing from our minds and hearts. Yet something will trigger a giggle and suddenly we see the humor in the sometimes desperate situations. As the years go by and life becomes even more interesting, it is important to remember, God still brings laughter and shouts of joy. It's all in how we view the circumstance.

A recent experience brought this to the forefront when both my husband and I were dealing with health issues. I was recovering from eye surgery and needed to be careful about bending, lifting, or any strenuous physical activity. Of course, that is the time when you seem to drop everything you touch—tissues, mail, papers, a book, cell phone. To make the scenario even more complicated, my husband could not help much due to his own health issues, so the floor remained cluttered. I finally figured out I could use the handy-dandy litter pickup tool we used for our front yard. It worked great—necessity is the mother of invention. So, I wandered through the house each day with my trusty picker-upper and was able to keep the floors clear. Score.

Immediately after my surgery, my husband ended up on crutches. An old knee injury had kicked in and he could barely put any weight on it. It had been bothering him, but he kept putting it off because of my eye surgery. I was scheduled for a post-op visit and he woke up that morning in pain. "I can still drive," he insisted. As long as he was seated, he was able to handle it. This was good, since I had a patch over my eye. I convinced him to drop me off at the eye doctor's office and to head directly to the ortho doctors who gave him a brace, crutches, and an appointment for an MRI.

I ended up calling my neighbors who came and rescued me from my eye doctor while my husband was at his own appointment. Arriving home before him, I looked out the window and saw him pull into our driveway. I grabbed a walking cane since I couldn't afford to trip and fall on our uneven brick sidewalk, being mindful of my eye recovery. He got out of the car and grabbed his new crutches. When I reached him, he balanced on one leg and handed me two more walking canes from the car. I couldn't help it. I started laughing and couldn't stop. We were all set for forward momentum with three walking canes and a pair of crutches. We presented quite the pathetic pair. Between the two of us, we certainly had enough medical devices to balance us out.

He caught the infectious laughter and joined in, so we both leaned on the car and couldn't stop laughing. We would start to straighten up, look at each other, and go off again on another wave of giddiness. Honestly, it felt good. Life had been stressful enough up to my surgery and I had been very concerned about it. Now to add to the picture, here I was looking like a one-eyed bandit and my husband on crutches limping around holding two other canes. The entire scene was comedic at best.

God filled our mouths with laughter that day. Shouts of joy? Well, yes. The Lord had answered many prayers during this time and I was joyful at a successful operation and already noticing clearer vision. We were thankful my husband now had crutches to take the weight off his knee and hopefully help it heal until they could run further tests. At least his pain level was now manageable. The days ahead would present many challenges, but between the two of us, we would stumble our way through and God would direct us, help us, strengthen us, and continue to fill our mouths with laughter, even at the most unexpected times.

There are moments I believe the Lord reaches down with heavenly feathers and tickles us until we have to succumb. We need our eyes open for the humor in life and to allow God to fill our mouth with laughter during these times. It is easy when circumstances are good, but even more special when we find laughter and joy when we least expect it. Only God.

prayer:

Lord, help us see the humor in the good times and the bad and to trust you have all situations in control. Show us how to recognize the funny times that happen each day, and to allow you to fill our mouths with laughter and to let your shouts of joy go forth.
In Jesus' name. Amen.

sassy suggestions:

» Physical limitations or aging issues may be trying, but they may also provide opportunities for laughter.

» Don't be afraid to laugh at yourself and your own human weaknesses.

» Rejoice in all the good times and believe there are good times in the future.

» Rejoice in the hard times and find the quirkiness of the current experience. Dig deep if you must, but find at least one thing *funny*.

» Help those around you to see the humor in everyday events.

36

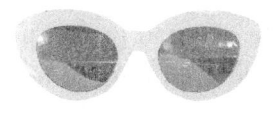

They will still bear fruit in old age, they will stay fresh and green (Psalm 92:14 NIV).

a season of harvest

Michelle Medlock Adams

Have you ever heard the metaphor that compares the different seasons of life to the four seasons of the year? In this comparison, the first quarter of life is spring, the second summer, the third autumn, and the fourth winter. After doing some quick math, you might realize that you're approaching that fourth quarter. You might be thinking … *Oh, great. Time to put on the ugly plastic snow boots and await the frigid winds of winter.*

But I don't believe it has to be that way. There's an old Jewish proverb that says, "For the ignorant, old age is winter. For the learned, it's a harvest." I love that idea, and the older I get, the more I understand the proverb's meaning. It's harvest time, baby!

Just think about what winter is like. Now, I absolutely love Christmastime. I'm that gal who goes all-out on my Christmas decorations. But man … when it's time to take down all the decorations and haul them back up into the attic, it's just depressing. The house looks empty, and it can feel that way, too, once all the relatives go back home to resume life as usual. In the months that follow, with gray skies, slushy roads, and nippy air, sometimes I don't even want to get out of bed. I just want to curl up under the covers and sleep through it all.

But harvest time? That's the time for bright colors and cozy weather. It's the time to make warm, tasty foods out of the crops that have been growing throughout the year. It's the time for Thanksgiving feasts shared with family—family that's grown after years of parenting and grand parenting.

Don't you want this season to be more like a harvest than a winter?

You see, it's all in how we approach this aging thing. We don't have to curl up under the covers and hide away in the dreary, cold, darkness of winter just because we are getting older. We don't have to spend our days thinking back on the warmth and fun of summer, longing to enjoy the sunshine again. If we look at this season as harvest time, then we can enjoy getting older and reap the benefits of all the wonderful seeds we've planted over the years.

Take a moment and think about your rich harvest. Maybe, after years of hard work raising children, you now enjoy spending time with grandchildren who fill your days with laughter and fun. Perhaps the many hours you invested in your career have enabled you to retire with enough money in the bank to enjoy life and travel without worrying about work. Maybe years of investing in relationships have yielded lifelong friends who share the same memories and have known you at every age and stage of life.

What attitude are you going to have about growing older? Are you going to get stuck in winter, convinced that all the good days have already passed? Or will you focus on all the blessings that your life has produced and enjoy these harvest years?

Spend some time with God and ask him to reveal the harvest that's yielded from your life's work. Reflect on the journey he has taken you on in order to create the life you have today. Some of the harvest may be obvious and bountiful. There may be other parts that have taken root, which are just about to bear fruit. Be expectant for that harvest.

And don't forget, it's never too late to plant new seeds, too. Different crops flourish in different seasons, and the same is true in many aspects of life. There's still time to accomplish important work on your terms. There's even more time for making new friends at this stage of life. Perhaps this season holds many new beginnings for you. While you enjoy your harvest, find new ideas and tasks to start cultivating. The seeds you plant now can bless you in your later years, as well as generations to come.

This isn't a season when everything in life dies and freezes over. It's not a season to hide under the blankets just to mourn the past. It's a season to harvest, enjoy the yield, and celebrate everything life has brought. Take a moment to be grateful for all God has grown through you and savor that harvest.

prayer:

Dear Lord, Thank you for all that you've planted in my life. You have been so generous to me. I ask you to reveal all that there is to harvest in this season, and I want you to know I am open to planting more seeds. Lead me in this season, Father. Please help me keep my eyes on the hope of the harvest, and not succumb to the dreariness of winter. In Jesus' mighty name. Amen.

sassy suggestions:

» Take note of all you are harvesting in this season. Trace each back through your life to see how God has been cultivating it over the years.

» Choose something new to plant in this season of life. It could be a relationship, a new job or hobby, a ministry, or something else God has put on your heart. Dutifully cultivate this new venture while you enjoy the harvest of others.

» Plant an actual plant and watch it grow. (I'm partial to succulents.) Use it as a beautiful reminder of what God has done in your life.

37

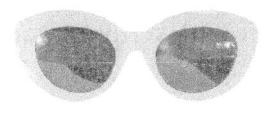

*Behold, thou hast made my days as an handbreadth;
and mine age is as nothing before thee...
(Psalm 39:5 KJV).*

five finger life

Cynthia A. Lovely

Spread out your fingers on one hand.

Even with longer fingers, this is a short measure. The distance in your hand span offers a profound reality—it is the measure of our days. Look again. Wow. We need to make each day count for Christ.

This eye-opening truth becomes more evident as we age and the days seem to fly by us. It is easy to look back and to wonder, *how we could possibly be this age. Surely there is a mistake.* The scripture in Psalms brings us great comfort and encouragement. "Mine age is as nothing before thee." Oh, I love this statement. If you are in your 50s or 60s and think the best part of your life is over, not true. Perhaps you are on a roller coaster ride into the 70s. No problem. Age is no hindrance to the Lord. No matter how old we are, we can move forward with confidence, anticipating new adventures in Christ. If there are doubts and fears about entering the *senior* phase and we start to believe the lie where our lives no longer matter or make a difference, we have this scripture stating the truth and putting to rest the lie of the enemy.

After all, age is just a number.

Of course, it may be a bit harder to accept once those numbers continue to climb. This shook me up one day while I was scrolling through social media. I came across a photo of a friend who was celebrating a landmark birthday. I admit I was impressed by the number. My immediate reaction was *Wow, she looks good for her age.*

On the heels of that statement, I sat up straighter as the thought clicked in my mind—she was only five years older than me. In five more years, it would be my face in that photo, claiming the important milestone. *Whoa.* The thought settled in my heart, along with the certainty I would not post a photo and reveal my age at any time. Just sayin.'

I had to laugh. Here I was thinking how good my senior friend looked at such an advanced age when I wasn't far behind her. Reading through her post, I was encouraged by her active ministry as a women's leader, pastor's wife, and also an author. Another example of ... age is as nothing before the Lord. Not to imply that he doesn't care about it, but the fact it will not hinder or negate the usefulness and influence of our lives. I think we can all breathe a sigh of relief here. Our value does not decrease with the increasing numerals and God will still use us for his purpose and his glory.

I also consider all those dear men and women who are much older and running circles around me in their ministries and effectiveness. They are an inspiration and encouragement. They have fought countless battles and learned invaluable lessons, standing strong in the knowledge and wisdom of God. I stand amazed at their energy level and all they manage to accomplish. Truly God has his hand of favor upon them and their age does not matter.

It is true not everyone has the same energy level or physical ability. Each person is different, and they face their own circumstances in the aging process. Some may be more able to accomplish certain tasks like my friend who posted her landmark photo. For others, it may be difficult if they face health issues and concerns. But if we are willing, God will continue to use us. He only looks for our availability.

My mother was a prime example. She struggled with health issues and limited means to accomplish much physically or socially. That did not stop her. She connected with pen pals through a magazine list. Soon she was corresponding with women all over the US, sharing her story of the goodness of God. I still have some of the letters sent to her. One letter expressed heartfelt thanks for helping this pen pal extend forgiveness to someone involved in her son's untimely death. What a miracle that my mother's written words would have this effect upon a complete stranger who became a friend through letters. Other notes showed clearly how my mother's writing ministry had touched their lives.

God has a plan and a purpose for our entire lives. There are always ways for God to use our gifts, talents, and skills which he has graciously bestowed upon us as long as we are willing. Remember to spread out those fingers and contemplate the shortness of life. It will kick into gear the importance of making every day count.

prayer:

God, we thank you that every one of our days matter to you. The rising numbers of our age do not surprise you or limit your ability to use us for your glory. Help us realize this and to continue to pursue you and your perfect will for our lives. In Jesus' name. Amen.

sassy suggestions:

- » Make a list of ideas you are still capable of doing to help others.
- » Reach out to people in your church community who would be blessed by a loyal friend.
- » Young people always need a good mentor and someone who genuinely cares for them.
- » Continue to work on your gifts and talents to reach a spirit of excellence in all you do.
- » Let go of any old grudges and/or resentments with others. Life is too short.

38

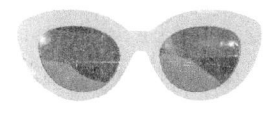

I have told you these things, so that in Me you may have (perfect) peace. In the world you have tribulation and distress and suffering, but be courageous (be confident, be undaunted, be filled with joy); I have overcome the world (My conquest is accomplished, My victory abiding)
(John 16:33 AMP).

victorious living

Connie Clyburn

Some days, it seems like tribulation and suffering take the form of getting in the slow lane at my local grocery store. How is it that no matter what day, time of day, and no matter what register line I'm in, it's always the one that drags along at a snail's pace?

Boy, does that make my blood pressure climb when I'm in a hurry. I do not like spending my time waiting in line. Basically, I don't enjoy waiting for anything. When I go to a restaurant, my hungry tummy is the only thing I can think about. If I go through a drive-thru, it's probably because I'm in a hurry to get somewhere else. Set me free already. Let me out of here so I can be on my way. Maybe, just maybe, if I took a breath and settled myself down, I could feel God nudging me to strike up a conversation with the person behind me in the grocery line who might need a kind word.

While I'm waiting at a restaurant, I can take advantage of that valuable time to socialize with those at my table. In the fast-food line, I could make a list of tasks that need to be done so I don't forget and cause more stress in my life (after putting my car in park, of course). Time waiting in line (or wherever) could be the down time I need to refocus my thoughts. When I take advantage of the slowdown, I notice the world around me.

I am, of course, being silly with my temporary and often imagined difficulties. Real distress, tribulation, and suffering are far worse than my grocery store lane frustrations. There are people living in destitute conditions in my country and around the world. I envision the homeless people in my own community having to sleep in cardboard boxes on the sidewalk. Tribulation seems far from me as I sit in my comfy house filled with all my favorite belongings and lie down in a warm bed.

Jesus is talking about anything that stresses us or causes us to lose our peace. He says there will be tribulation in this life. He has already overcome every plan of the enemy that dares to discombobulate. Jesus' death on the cross provided the way of salvation and so much more. It gives us all we need to live victoriously in this life—joy, strength, and health.

Walking in victory enables us to live the life he intends. If we're broke, busted, and disgusted, how can we fulfill God's plan? He needs us to stay in the game. Yes, I said God *needs* us. It's His plan to work through us mere mortals. If we stay strong and able, and believing God's Word, we will be ready to help carry out his plan on the earth. The Bible shows us multiple examples of God working through people to accomplish his plans.

It is easy to get caught up in the frustrations of this life. When it seems there's not enough budget to cover expenses or work gets under your skin, take a breath, and remember that Jesus has your back. He said that he came to give us abundant life. He wants to work with you and through you as you live out life in victory. And what's better than being an active part of God's plan?

Be courageous, Jesus commands. He says this several times throughout the New Testament. If it were not possible to accomplish, he wouldn't have included it in his admonitions. And it is possible to accomplish because we get our courage from him. In his earthly ministry, Jesus faced the angry crowds, the Pharisees, and even death for us. The ultimate reason was to give us eternal life, but he also walked through all those circumstances, taking on the worst of the worst, so we could be victorious in life. It's not a victory to be hidden away behind closed doors for a special occasion. It's a victory to be used every day. Courage to be victorious causes us to live in peace all the time.

prayer:

Dear Lord, Thank you for setting the example for me to follow as I live out my life. You showed me what courage looks like. You lived a victorious life so that I could experience victory. I see, now, that I can be successful and live out the plan you've set before me. I know you will be with me every step of the way. In Jesus' name. Amen.

sassy suggestions:

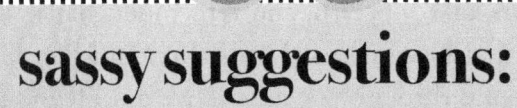

» **Gospel truth** – refresh your mind by studying Jesus' earthly ministry as detailed in the Gospels and how he overcame the world for us.

» **Thankfulness** – Being thankful will help you focus on God's goodness

» **Praise** – Praising the Lord always helps lift your mood

» **Party.** – Celebrate every achievement and thank God for his divine favor on your life.

» **Togetherness** – Plan outings with special friends and family. Even a coffee date now and again will help keep the ties that bind hearts held tight.

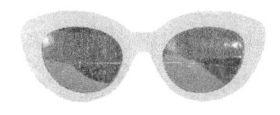

But those who trust in the LORD will find new strength. They will soar high on wings like eagles. They will run and not grow weary. They will walk and not faint (Isaiah 40:31 NLT).

the final category

Michelle Medlock Adams

a couple of years ago, while visiting friends in Texas, I attended a church near Tyler. After being greeted quite warmly, an usher asked me to fill out a guest card and place it into the offering plate. As I wrote down all my pertinent information, my eyes settled on the age boxes—Under 12, 12-17, 18-29, 30-44, and 45-over.

No way. I am actually in the final age category? The oldest group. The end of the line. How did this happen? When did this happen?

So many questions, and apparently, so little time left to ponder them. I had a hard time focusing on what the minister shared after realizing I had now been defined as old—insert huge lump in my throat.

I guess I knew I was *over 45*, but I hadn't realized what being over 45 actually meant until that moment. Know what I mean? Seeing it in black and white made that fact much more real for me.

Though math is not my strong suit, I began doing some quick addition. That's when it hit me—I had probably lived more years on this earth than I had left to live. *Oh, my gosh. How did this happen without me being keenly aware of the magnitude of the situation?* At first, the truth literally took my breath away. But after the initial shock wore off, I had clarity. I had a moment. You know, one of those moments that you'll remember the rest of your life.

In that moment, my heart cried out to the Lord, "God, don't let me waste any of the years I have left on this earth. Help me live them with direction—divine direction—purpose and passion."

You see, I thought my trip to Texas was to meet with clients, learn from amazing writers in my new non-fiction tribe, take promotional shots for my upcoming *Dinosaur Devotions* book, help lead a Serious Writer Tour Stop, and spend time with some of my favorite, lifelong friends. And it was … it was all that, but it was so much more. It was a chance to reconnect with myself and recommit my life to God's plans for the rest of my life.

Today, as I write this devotion, I'm still over 45. I didn't wake up at age 30 again, but you know what? I don't even desire that anymore. Sure, I'll still be using anti-aging skincare (the best I can afford), drinking lots of water and fewer Polar Pops, and working out as often as my schedule allows, but I've realized the most important part of growing old gracefully is knowing who you are and *whose* you are. It's waking up every day with a heart full of thankfulness and an excitement that God isn't through with me yet. I have a sticky note on my laptop that says, "You're not too old, and it's not too late." And that's what I want to remind you of today. So what if we're in that final age category. We're still here, and we still have a lot of life left in us. I hope this serves as an *a-ha moment* for you.

Spend some time with your heavenly Father and allow him to give you direction for this season of your life. No matter how old you are, what you've been through, or what you're going through right now, God has a plan, a purpose, and a perfect peace just waiting for you to unwrap. Remember, God's timing is always perfect, and this is his time. This is his time to work through you to accomplish the great and mighty. So, be excited. God isn't through with us yet, and his Word says he will renew our strength. We will run and not grow weary. So, lace up those leopard tennis shoes and run your race. I'll run mine, and we'll finish strong together.

prayer:

Dear Lord, Help me to fulfill every plan you have for my life. And, Father, help me be grateful and joyful as we take this journey together. I give my fears to you, Lord, and trade them in for new fire, increased energy, and a love for life that I've never had before. Thank you, God, for this wake-up call today.
In Jesus' name. Amen.

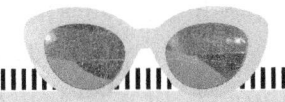

sassy suggestions:

» Do something every day that inches you closer to a dream God has placed in your heart. Working toward your dreams will keep you motivated.

» Get an accountability partner to keep you on track to achieving your dreams, walking in your calling, and moving forward with excitement. Have weekly check-ins with each other, pray for each other, and encourage one another.

» Get your focus on God and off of your age. As simple as that sounds, it will make a profound difference in your life. Meditate on his over 7,000 promises found in the Bible. Let his Word remind you of who you are in Christ Jesus. Here are two scriptures to get you started.

» "For we are his workmanship, created in Christ Jesus for good works, which God prepared beforehand, that we should walk in them" (Ephesians 2:10 ESV).

» "But you are a chosen race, a royal priesthood, a holy nation, a people for his own possession, that you may proclaim the excellencies of him who called you out of darkness into his marvelous light" (1 Peter 2:9 ESV).

40

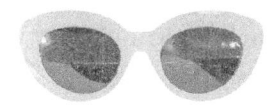

*Do not store up for yourselves treasures on earth,
where moths and vermin destroy,
and where thieves break in and steal
(Matthew 6:19 NIV).*

scrooge thieves

Cynthia A. Lovely

I raced out of my office to my car outside, a burst of adrenaline kicking in at the disturbing news. Someone had broken into our sweet country home.

Reminding myself of the fact treasures on earth fade away brought some measure of comfort. Add to that the fact no one was home at the time of the break-in, so no one was hurt in the process. Thank God. However, it was still unsettling and I didn't know what I would find when I got there.

I prayed all the way home, knowing my husband was on his way to meet me there. A police car was in our driveway since the theft had already been reported and the police officer escorted me inside. Belongings were thrown about willy-nilly and I was admonished not to touch anything. It looked like a quick job since they had already hit other houses in the neighborhood and were pushing their luck by continuing the thievery. We had felt safe here for many years and never had any problems like this before, which made it all the more disturbing.

When I went upstairs to our bedroom and found drawers pulled out and objects scattered, it hit me hard. They had invaded our privacy and ransacked our home. It left me with a vulnerable feeling of violation and loss. We got through the day with the help of the town policemen and prayers of friends and family. We had to list what had been taken, but the good news was they had caught the thieves and all our stolen items were still in their vehicle. Yes, God was watching out for us.

We don't possess valuable jewelry or expensive electronics, but they stole both our laptops and all our wrapped Christmas presents. A writer's worst nightmare—a stolen laptop with all my years of writings on it. Now that hurt. When we were finally allowed in the police station and I identified my laptop, I cried. Saved. We had to wait a few weeks for our items to be released to us, but the kind judge allowed us to take our Christmas gifts back in time for the holiday.

Even in the midst of the turmoil and strife after the break-in, we were thankful for God's grace. The damage to our house was minimal. The front door and locks had to be replaced with deadbolts and belongings had to be re-organized as they threw so much around during the theft. This experience put a whole new slant on our material possessions. How true it is that our real possessions are not material belongings on this earth.

My husband and I have discussed this before. What would we grab first if a fire started at our house? Of course, his first answer is ...

me, but it is a close call to his saxophone. I guess I'll be sure to stay close to his sax if a fire breaks out. I would, in turn, be most concerned for his safety. Next, I would probably grab my laptop along with memory boxes or photos and any personal records. So when it comes down to it, we don't really have many treasures here on this earth.

As we grow older and the tendency may be to hold on to *things*, perhaps it is time to re-evaluate our possessions and pare down our belongings. The minimalist lifestyle is looking better and better. Like the scripture states, thieves may break in and steal or the treasures may be destroyed by moths and vermin. This is certainly true for us, since we live in the country with a continual battle of insects and critters.

I don't want to follow the crowd and desire more and more of the material. There is always a new iPhone better than the last one, a larger monitor screen to watch more movies on, and a classier and more impressive car to drive. Yet when our home was broken into, all that truly mattered was that my husband and I were both safe and no one was harmed. The robbery brought it all into perspective.

I am grateful for all God has given us. He always provides our needs and even some of our wants. But our hope, our joy, our life is in him. In truth, no one can steal Jesus, our treasure, from us. The Scrooge thieves may have tried to steal Christmas from us, but they could not steal the treasure in our hearts.

prayer:

Lord, you and you alone are the greatest gift of all. We thank you for providing our needs and we ask for wisdom to keep our focus on you. We don't want to be consumed with treasures of earth but to build up our treasures of heaven. In Jesus' name. Amen.

sassy suggestions:

» **If you had to move out of your home, think about what you need to keep and what you are willing to let go. Pare down and donate items.**

» **Now consider all the treasures in heaven you want to build up. Treasures like helping those around you in your daily walk with God and becoming open to the needs of others.**

» **List other ways you can do this, such as committing your prayer time and Bible study to grow deeper in your walk with the Lord.**

» **Support your pastor and church family in the work of God.**

» **Give your tithes and offerings to your local congregation, church plants, and missionaries.**

41

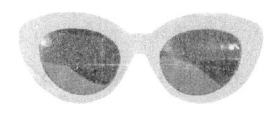

Little children (believers, dear ones), you are of God and you belong to Him and have (already) overcome them (the agents of the antichrist); because He who is in you is greater than he (Satan) who is in the world (of sinful mankind) (1 John 4:4 AMP).

defeating giants

Connie Clyburn

God is greater than the giants I face. They can puff up until they look big and scary, but it's just an act. The giants that try to stand against us are no match for our God.

The giants of this world's system often come at me, trying to defeat me. Just like Goliath did with David in the Old Testament, they taunt and yell in defiance of my God. They proudly challenge my God-given dreams, telling me I'll never amount to anything. Their shouts try to tear down and destroy. I've held on to those dreams planted in my heart so long that in some cases, it can feel like they're slipping away into the abyss of the *what ifs* and *forget it, it will never happen*. It's never too late for the dreams God has placed in my heart. He will finish the good work he started in me.

The truth is, I already have the victory through Jesus who has overcome the giants for me. The power to trample over them is mine because Jesus has already defeated the enemy. I can stand strong knowing God's Word promises he is faithful to perform what he's put in my heart. If I keep moving forward, reaching for the goal, he will be right there with me, ensuring my success.

That doesn't stop the giants from rearing their ugly heads. They will try to show up. I've held onto the dream of being a full-time writer for years, planning to see it come to fruition someday. Then the giants of *you're not relevant, you're a nobody,* and *no one wants to read what you have to say* fling their insults at me. I remind them my God is bigger. I encourage myself in the Lord, dwelling on the truth of that verse. "Greater is He that is in me than he that is in the world." God declares me victorious over every ugly dart shot my way.

Many years ago, a mere week out of college with the ink still fresh on my degree, I started my writing career as a newspaper reporter. The work was rewarding, but life changes soon sent me in different directions. Along the way, I abandoned newspaper writing and floated through career changes that were far from the profession for which I'd trained. I did a little writing here and there, but full-time jobs didn't leave me much time or energy for much else. Then something sparked the writing bug in me anew. I remembered going on assignments, writing about people and their interesting lives. I realized how much I'd loved meeting them and telling their stories. I missed it.

Spring forward to present day. I now have a blog, authored and published a children's book, and co-authored the book you're holding. I believe it's what God meant for me to do all along, though I didn't understand that at first. So here I am, a bit (ahem) older and wiser. As I write this, I'm planning to retire from the job I've held for the last 20+ years. Is it too late to pursue more of my dreams? No way. I have more fun ideas and plans than ever and I've gained a lot of knowledge that I didn't have as a younger me. I think the timing is perfect.

Take heart, the timing is perfect for you too. You're poised on the edge of the most exciting time of life. It's time—go for it. Don't wait any longer. Taking a quote from a popular Bible teacher–"Do it afraid".

God will continue to point you in the direction of his plans for your life if you keep putting one foot in front of the other. He won't make you do what you're supposed to do, but he will work with you as you go along. He has already prepared the road ahead. He will also walk along with you, and he doesn't expect you to do it alone. You can't do it by yourself. Reread the stories of heroes and heroines of the Old and New Testaments. All of them were able to do great accomplishments by and through God's help and strength.

Starting with a small step can help unlock the door to an avalanche of prospects. One move forward is progress in the right direction.

prayer:

Dear Lord, Thank you for encouraging me through your Word. You enable me to conquer anything the enemy throws at me. You are in me and I'm in you. Use me, God, for your divine purposes. I dedicate my talents, abilities, and my time to you.
In Jesus' name. Amen.

sassy suggestions:

» Let your dreams soar. It's possible to realize your goals at any age. Greater is he that is in you.

» How old will you be in 5, 10, 20 years if you pursue your dreams—the same age you'll be if you don't.

» Consider the lives you'll touch as you go after the purposes God put you on earth to accomplish.

» Nothing is too big with God on your side, enabling you to trample over ferocious looking giants in his name.

42

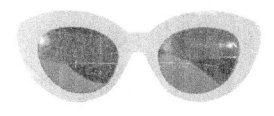

*Be very careful, then, how you live—not as unwise but as wise, making the most of every opportunity, because the days are evil
(Ephesians 5:15–16 NIV).*

rejoice in life

Michelle Medlock Adams

As secretary of my graduating class, one responsibility that has stuck with me over the years is helping plan our high school reunions. This year marked 35 years (Class of 1987, baby.) I was so excited to gather everyone together again and see what people had been up to, share pictures of our grandbabies, and reminisce about our many high school shenanigans.

As our committee began reaching out to all 378 members of our graduating class, excitement quickly turned to sadness when we discovered far too many of our classmates had passed on. Where did the time go? And wouldn't it have been nice to see those classmates at least one more time?

You know, the older you get, the more keenly aware you become that death is inevitable. You start losing more and more people who are special to you, and you notice how much closer your own age creeps toward the average life expectancy. I remember the first time I realized I had probably lived more years than I had left to live. I was depressed for a week. I was officially *freaked out*. Maybe you've experienced those same feelings.

It seems many people reach retirement age and begin seeing the world through a *why bother* filter. Do you know people like that? They avoid trying to do anything new. They let the challenges that come with aging stop them from living life. They don't believe there's much left for them on earth, so they start longing for heaven. Maybe you know someone who falls into that group, or maybe you actually fit that description.

Well, I've got good news for you. Whether you just attended your 35th high school reunion or your 60th, God is not done with you yet. Sure, you can look forward to spending eternity in heaven with the Lord, but you shouldn't spend so much time longing, that you have no time for living. Be excited that God has more days planned for you. Be grateful he can still use you to accomplish big tasks while you're here on this earth because time passes quickly. That's why Paul wrote, in his letter to the Ephesians, "the days are evil." Time can so easily slip by, and we shouldn't take any of it for granted.

When I think about the years I have left, I am no longer freaked out. I choose to live out my full days here on earth, pursuing God's callings and loving those around me. I don't dread death. Instead, I look to the future with hope in Jesus. In other words, I don't dwell on death. I rejoice in life.

So, if you are living with the *just waiting to die* mentality—it's time to snap out of it. If God has given you another day, use it for his glory. Focus your attention on what you *are* still able to do instead of what you are not. Get a new attitude. There's life left to live. Live each day with intention. Trust me, you have a lot left to offer. You wouldn't still be here if God didn't have a plan for the rest of your life, so stop longing for heaven and begin living with purpose.

prayer:

Dear Lord, Thank you for giving me this day on earth. I look forward to eternity with you, but I won't let that keep me from spending today with you as well. Please show me the plans you still have for me, Lord, and give me the strength to fulfill them before my days on earth are through. In Jesus' name. Amen.

sassy suggestions:

» **Start a gratitude journal.** Every day, list three things you are grateful for on that particular day.
» **Ask God what new venture he might have for you** during this season of your life. Start brainstorming and pray over each idea.
» **Get social.** One of the best ways to get out of a funk is by talking with other people. Join a Bible study at your church, start a hobby group, or have a family video call.

43

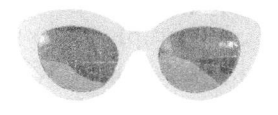

The apostles gathered around Jesus and reported to him all they had done and taught. Then, because so many people were coming and going that they did not even have a chance to eat, he said to them, "Come with me by yourselves to a quiet place and get some rest"
(Mark 6:30-31 NIV).

naptime

Cynthia A. Lovely

doing and teaching, people coming and going, no chance to eat or rest. This statement strikes a chord of familiarity and could easily relate to our current chaotic lives.

It sounds like busy days back then and perhaps a forerunner of Christian ministry today. The apostles were caught up doing and teaching and the crowds kept coming until Jesus admonished them to come away with him to rest. There are times we also become busy in the work of God and we forget the need for a quiet place. God calls us away from our schedules to find a cozy corner of relaxation.

I've often chatted with friends who have retired. They inform me their schedule is more hectic than ever. Hmm … it makes me wonder. We may have convinced ourselves we are not truly valuable or successful unless we can complain about how many items we are juggling. It is not bad to be busy. Yet, there is a balance between pursuing goals and always seeking more with finding time for yourself to rest and draw new strength to carry on. This brings us to that little three letter word—nap.

Love this word. Even the sound of it is appealing—short, sweet, and calming. Most people would welcome an occasional nap. It is amusing how when we were young children and had to be set down for a nap, we sometimes fought against it. I recall long ago when I was in school, probably kindergarten, where we had a scheduled nap time every day. We each had our own little throw rug to curl up on for our afternoon siesta. The background sounds of the low voice of the teacher admonishing a student to hush, the giggles of those kids who just did not want to be quiet and the eventual wave of drowsiness coming over the group as we all slid into dreamland. Lovely childhood innocence wrapped up in our nap times.

In remembering those days, I can't help but think at this current stage of life; how I would love for someone to make me go lay down and take a nap. Because this probably won't happen, I have to make the decision myself when I tire out in the late afternoon. The roomy couch filled with comfy cushions beckons me. I grab a leopard print furry throw and curl up. Ahh. I tuck in and the afternoon quiet lulls me to sleep. Delicious. There are times my body craves this naptime and I've learned not to fight it. Sweet slumber mid-day can be refreshing and renewing and give new energy for the rest of the day. It is not wimping out or causing us to be less effective in our pursuits. On the contrary, it enables us to move forward and complete more endeavors and meet more goals.

It is a comfort to know Jesus saw the human needs and admonished his apostles to come away to a quiet space and rest. Often in this place of stillness, we drift away into the assurance he is watching over us. Just as our teachers watched over us in our afternoon naps and our parents kept an eye on us as we napped at home, Jesus watches over us as we obey his instruction and find a time of rest. In those calm, slumbering moments, I believe he draws near to us and restores and renews us while we nap.

Feeling sleepy today? Go ahead, take a nap. I realize if you are working full-time, this might not be an option. Your boss may not understand the value of afternoon naps. So on the weekends, give yourself this luxury when you feel naptime is calling your name. It doesn't have to be long, a short rest is still advantageous. There will be times when we can go without it, but sooner or later in this crazy and nonstop culture, you will probably need a nap.

prayer:

Lord, thank you for seeing our need for rest and renewal. Help us recognize and respond to your calling away. And thank you that you come away with us and watch over us as we rest. Revive us and restore us. In Jesus' name. Amen.

sassy suggestions:

» It is wise to have a plan set up for naptime. Not structured too tightly, but mapped out enough to know it is a possibility when you begin to droop and fade out later in the day. If you are a list person, you may even pencil it in on your schedule.

» The first decision is to find the best time to nap. This may vary from your day-to-day activities, so it is smart to stay flexible. Choose a quiet part of the day when the neighborhood is peaceful. Maybe shut off your phone or at least turn down the volume.

» Next, choose the location. For some people, a couch is the ideal place. With plenty of soft pillows and a cozy throw, a short snooze can work wonders. Others may like to doze off in a recliner or a comfortable armchair. Figure out what works best for you.

» There are others who drift towards their bed for a deeper slumber. I tend to avoid this since it is easier to nod off for too long. I keep the bedroom for night sleep unless I am really exhausted or not feeling well. If that is the situation, then I give myself permission for a longer snooze. After you choose your ideal time and place, enjoy your afternoon siesta and awake refreshed and productive for the rest of your day.

44

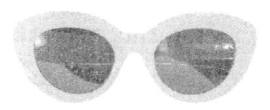

He who dwells in the shelter of the Most High will remain secure and rest in the shadow of the Almighty (whose power no enemy can withstand) (Psalm 91:1 AMP).

dwell and rest

by Connie Clyburn

I had good intentions. My daily plan sounded good—do everything on my to-do list as soon as my feet hit the floor. But first, coffee. Then sit down at the computer and turn into a writing dynamo. My well-crafted plans always seem to melt into the quickly passing morning hours somewhere between reading everyone's a.m. greetings on social media, wishing every dog on Facebook "Happy Birthday" and making sure I post birthday greetings for all my human friends. Because, you know, that's a requirement or my day won't be complete.

I'm so easily distracted. There, I said it. It's easy to get caught up in doing it all—being there, picking up, cleaning up, caring for people, caring for the dog, feeding the barn cats … the list goes on and on. In fact, it kind of feels weird when there's nothing to do. I get a little antsy and don't know what to do with myself.

Social media is a habit that I could (and should) cut back on viewing. Even if I don't have photos to post of my own dog eating breakfast, I scroll through the other pics and read about all that's going on in the outside world and then get sucked into the drama like Barbara Eden being sucked back into her bottle in *I Dream of Jeannie*. On one hand, it lets me know how to pray for others who are facing difficulties, but I get so caught up in the action going on in other's lives. I have learned not to read the comments on my friends' posts. Everybody has an opinion about every little topic, from how to open a can of peas properly to what to feed your dog.

I think I'm addicted to engagement—participating in the busyness of life. I don't even have to be physically active at the time. Lying in bed at night planning the next day's activities seems perfectly normal. Remembering to set my alarm just so I can keep up with all that needs to be done the next day is not out of my ordinary. I want to be ready right out of the gate. Where does it stop?

Hold up a minute, sista. Whew, I'm ready to take a nap just thinking about it (probably from lying in bed at night watching the *Golden Girls* while making out my to-do list). I need to take a break.

I slow down and take a deep breath. I feel my rapidly beating heart settle down a notch or two. I let God do what only he can. Yes, I have a part, but what is it?

Then I hear him say, "I'm glad you asked."

"Read Psalm 91 in my Word again, but slower this time," he gently nudges me.

He who dwells in the shelter ... will remain secure and rest....

My part is dwelling and resting in his presence. Not being busy, not taking care of something or somebody, not running out to the store. There's nothing wrong with doing any of that. I must slow down and recognize the Lord wants to take care of all the concerns of my life. He wants to do the same for you.

We're to dwell in and soak up each moment. Relish life. Dwell and rest while filling up the grocery buggy or stopping by to pick up pizza for dinner. Rest in knowing our God is holding us and he can (and will) handle anything going on in our lives.

I'm getting it. The lightbulbs in my head might be slowly going on one at a time instead of the whole string glowing together at once. The idea is to trust and rest.

prayer:

Dear Lord, Thank you for **getting** *me. There are days I struggle to make sense of the busyness. You don't shame me or yell at me. You gently remind me through your Word that my part is simply to dwell and rest in you. Your plan is perfect. Help me follow the way you've prepared for me to walk. Thank you, Lord, for your immense love and acceptance. I love being in your inner circle that's quiet and restful. There, I am refreshed, and my joy is renewed. I love you.*
In Jesus' name. Amen.

sassy suggestions:

» **Morning quiet time** – while stumbling to the kitchen to start the coffee, meditate on the goodness of God and how he is always with you. He is there while you sleep at night, when you walk out to get the paper, even while the coffee is brewing.

» **Rainy day?** While sipping your coffee or tea, dwell in the beauty of the rain that waters the grass and provides for the animals.

» **On a clear day**, get outside and enjoy that sunshine. Take a walk and consider how even the sun's rays are for your benefit. The sun provides essential vitamins that your body needs to function properly. That's pretty amazing.

» **Starry, starry night.** Personally, it's my favorite time to sky gaze. Look into the night at all the neat sights. Find planets that are visible in whatever season it is or pick out constellations. Dwell in the assurance that the One who created them has you in the palm of his mighty hand.

» **Thankfulness.** Being thankful gets your mind focused on the goodness of God and off the issues of the day. I find it helpful to take a few minutes to make a list of blessings. I can keep adding to it and it's always there to refer to time and time again.

45

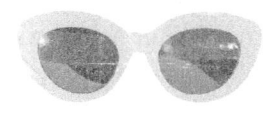

I will both lie down in peace, and sleep; For You alone, O Lord, make me dwell in safety (Psalm 4:8 NKJV).

lullaby and good night

Cynthia A. Lovely

3 am. The bright numbers of the digital clock mock me. I close my eyes, hoping to drift off into a peaceful slumber. The day before, it was 1:30 am when my eyes popped open. I toss, I turn, rearrange the pillow for the umpteenth time. The struggle is real.

I consider getting up, but I know it will make it even harder to go back to sleep. Somewhere along the way, my internal time clock skewed and I haven't found a way to reset it.

I turn my mind towards scriptures. I remember the advice to *lie down in peace*, yet I know there were troubling thoughts and concerns of the day that lingered. I guess I entertained a parade of worries when I didn't fall asleep right away. I wondered if I would meet my next deadline. I forgot to check on my friend who was quarantined. There was that weird noise the car had been making and the concern of another repair bill. Hmm … I could not solve any of these problems at 3 am.

The running list of concerns did not help my state of mind or create a restful atmosphere. I needed to give it all over to the Lord so the troubles wouldn't multiply in the recesses of my mind. God is the only One who makes me "dwell in safety." Yet here I am again in the early hours, waiting for sleep to overtake me. I don't want to face the truth, but I'm thinking this is probably yet another sign of growing older.

Facing this reality, I determine to hold on to the scriptures and settle the Word of God in my heart and in my spirit. God has promised us peace and rest as we look to him. During the early morning hours when I wake unexpectedly, perhaps this is a call to prayer. Maybe this is a time where I am still and quiet and the outside noise is gone. The Lord has my attention. I'm not going to pick up a cell phone or check for any messages. The only important message, at this time, is from him. I thank God for his unending blessings. I think of all those in need of prayer and bring their names before the throne of God.

When I get through the list, I go over comforting scriptures and focus on peaceful songs of worship. These thoughts bring me to sweet memories of my mother rocking me to sleep in her old rocker, singing soft lullabies to her little girl. I can still hear her voice and feel the calming effect of the rhythm. A time when I was a young child, held securely in mother's arms, lulled by the motion of the rocker and cozy in the warm comfort of her embrace.

Yes, that is the image of our Lord holding us in his arms and singing over us, with a love that surpasses all others. And oh, what security and safety we find in his arms.

Inspired by this image, I pen a lullaby in my head. "Lord, place your hand upon my brow, whisper words of comfort now. Hold me close throughout the night until the morning light. Cover me with peace and rest. Touch me with your gentleness. Take away my every fear. Dear Lord, draw near."

Ah … the peace that passes all understanding. I can almost feel his gentle hand upon my brow and hear his tender words of love. I sing it to myself softly so as not to awaken my slumbering husband. My eyes drift shut once again and restorative sleep returns.

I'm sure there are many remedies for insomnia and sleeplessness, and some are safer than others. I'm not into medications, but I know there are more natural solutions with diet, vitamins and melatonin. These methods may be beneficial to a point. However, the safest, surest, most wonderful answers to sleep problems are still found in God's Word and the comfort of his dear presence. If you are troubled with interrupted sleep all out of kilter, turn it over to Jesus and rest secure in him. Pray, recite scripture, go over slow worship choruses and before you know it…zzzz. Sweet dreams.

prayer:

Dear Lord, as I lay down to rest, cover me with your gentle peace and help me relax in the comfort of your safety. In Jesus' name. Amen.

sassy suggestions:

» Take a little time to prepare before you go to sleep at night. There are simple ways to decrease broken and interrupted sleep patterns. Chill out a few hours before and find a pattern that works for your schedule.

» Avoid all caffeine late in the day. This includes any coffee, tea or that tempting piece of chocolate.

» No electronics for at least an hour or two before you sleep. You don't need scrolling images of social media floating through your thoughts—way too distracting. And the *blue light* can work against your sleep.

» Keep the bedroom at a comfortable temperature, not too hot or too cold. If your spouse loves it cold and you're freezing, let him use a personal fan aimed in his direction while you snuggle under the covers.

» Pull down the shades so no disturbing light pours into the room. Block any electronic devices with their blinking lights or any hallway night light that may shine too brightly into the bedroom. Sleep well. Be at peace.

46

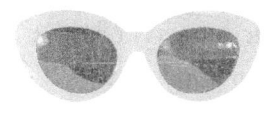

Then Jesus, knowing they were going to come and take Him by force to make Him king, withdrew again to the mountainside by Himself (John 6:15 AMP).

the mountains are calling

Connie Clyburn

Jesus headed for the hills when circumstances got hairy. I can relate to that. This world gets to be a little much sometimes with all that's going on around us. Voices are everywhere giving their opinions, whether or not I asked for them. If Jesus needed an occasional break, it makes sense that I would also need to retreat sometimes.

A true retreat refreshes and restores. It provides time to logout, unplug, and look at life from a new perspective. Lush, tree-lined mountains offer inviting places for a simple retreat. A mountain emanates an ethereal feeling, inviting me to discover secret places and hidden treasures worth seeking out—every leafy trail bids the explorer in me to investigate. The reward at the end of the trail is the spectacular view. Nature provides amazing vistas and cozy nooks to spend time talking to our heavenly Father.

One of my favorite places to visit is the Breaks Interstate Park, with its rolling mountain tops that spill over from Virginia into Kentucky. The anticipation will never grow old, no matter how many times I drive the winding backwoods road leading up the mountain. As soon as I see the park's welcome sign, my heart skips. There, I am cradled between craggy peaks wrought by mighty hands. Any troubles tumbling in my mind ease into peace. One night when I stayed there on a work trip, a storm came up and the power went out. I watched from the sliding glass door as flashes of lightning danced across the dark mountain range, reminding me that God shelters me.

The things of this world will try to take me by force, like an angry mob on a mission. There's no need to fear because my protector is here. He sweeps me up into the mountain of his care, where he provides a quiet place to refocus.

Life can be overwhelming. It's easy to get a little lost in an increasingly loud world that constantly competes for our attention. Oh, but a visit to the mountainside can set the mind straight and help it regain focus. When Jesus physically walked this earth, he was all God, but he was also all man. As the scriptures show, he had to take breaks to get alone to pray and remember his mission. Many times, he chose a hillside or a mountainside to hide away. I find it interesting that Jesus often chose a place in nature to get away from the noise of the crowd. It reminds me of a scene in a movie about Jesus' ministry on earth. In this scene, Jesus came walking back into camp one evening where the disciples and others waited for him. Jesus looked worn and weathered from working with the crowds he had, no doubt, been teaching and healing all day. Instead of gathering around the fire to talk, Jesus bid them all good night without saying much. One woman took off his sandals to wash his feet and legs. That interaction impacted me. It reminded me Jesus wasn't an *energizer bunny* who could go, go, go without ever taking a break.

We can learn from this simple yet profound lesson. Where else can we see the hand of God more clearly than in nature? The vibrant feathers of various birds testify to our amazing Creator. Intricate patterns woven in the petals of a wildflower shout *there is a God who cares about me.* Walk into a grove of trees or even out into your own backyard. Get quiet, close your eyes and listen. In the evening, crickets and tree frogs chirp out their nighttime song. Mornings feature a chorus of birds welcoming the day. Step outside just after a rain shower. Breathe deeply and smell the heavy scent of woody tree bark, fresh green grass, and the sweet fragrance of the wildflowers. He created it all for you to enjoy.

God knew we would need times of solace—something to help us regain focus and remind us to slow down. His message, "Come retreat to the mountain with me." Thanks Father, I think I'll do just that.

prayer:

Dear Lord, Thank you for times of refreshing. Lead me into quiet retreats where I'm reminded of your personal love and care. Help me escape the noisy crowds where I can hear only your still, quiet voice. Thank you for shepherding me in the way I need to go.
In Jesus' name. Amen.

sassy suggestions:

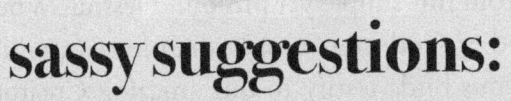

» **Run away to the mountains.** Book a cabin or a room at a secluded inn for a few days of rest and relaxation.

» **No time to hop in the car and run away to the mountains?** Visit the neighborhood park. There's at least one park in your community. If you live out in the country, even better, the back roads provide a solace all their own.

» **Maybe you live in the middle of a bustling city.** Find a corner coffee shop and sit at an outside table. You'll be surprised at the sounds of nature you can hear in the city.

» **Turn your bedroom into a retreat** by opening a window, then wake up to a chorus of chirps to enjoy nature in spring, summer and fall depending on where you live (maybe not in winter when the temps are low).

» **Home Base**—steal away with your Bible to a quiet porch corner or anywhere you can get quiet and enjoy being outside.

47

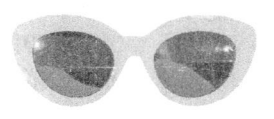

"For I know the plans I have for you," says the LORD. "They are plans for good and not for disaster, to give you a future and a hope" (Jeremiah 29:11 NLT).

never too late

Michelle Medlock Adams

do you sometimes feel like the best part of your life is already over? Like you've missed out on dreams you had because you didn't accomplish them when you were younger? Unfortunately, these regrets aren't uncommon, and they can cause very real and very intense dissatisfaction. There have been studies that show the older a person gets, the more likely depression will happen. But we don't have to let the same happen to us.

We all have dreams we haven't realized. Maybe it's a career you never started, a degree you never finished, or a project you never tackled. But here's the deal—it's not too late. You haven't missed the boat. Your age does not limit the calling God has for your life. He has big plans for you, even still.

A beautiful example of this is Susan Boyle. For much of her life, she spent her days living in the Scottish countryside, taking care of her aging mother and her cat, and volunteering at her church. She had always dreamed of becoming a professional singer. So, at

47, she auditioned for "Britain's Got Talent." (You can watch her initial audition online, and I highly recommend it.) As she stepped out onto the stage, you could see the confusion on the audience's faces. *What's this frumpy old lady doing up on the stage? Is she for real?*

But the moment Susan opened her mouth, everything changed. As she sang the first lyrics of *I Dreamed a Dream*, the crowd erupted in applause. Her astounding performance went viral and advanced her to the final rounds of the competition. After her success on the show, she released an album, which hit number one on the Billboard 200 in the United States and became the UK's best-selling debut album of all time.

And that's not all. A couple of years ago, she shared in an interview that she had always wanted to have children. So, at the age of 58, she decided to look into fostering. Susan has never stopped dreaming, and she pursues her dreams in a big way. Susan isn't the only one. Many world changers were late bloomers. Beloved author Laura Ingalls Wilder didn't publish her first book until she was 65, and her books are still childhood favorites nearly a century later. Grandma Moses didn't start painting until she was 76, and even with no art schooling or training, her work is now of historic importance. Sarah, in the Bible, didn't have her first son until she was 90, and that son became a patriarch of the Jewish nation. She had given up, but God hadn't.

What dream has God given to you? Is it to write a book? Is it to teach a bible study? Is it to start your own business?

What is holding you back? In 2 Peter 1:10–11, Peter wrote, "Therefore, my brothers and sisters, make every effort to confirm your calling and election. For if you do these thigns, you will never stumble, and you will receive a rich welcome into the eternal kingdom of our Lord and Savior Jesus Christ." (NIV) If God is calling you to a dream, you should pursue it.

There's no need for you to sit around and regret the dreams you haven't accomplished. Instead, rekindle that dream inside of you and ask God to open the doors for you according to his perfect timing. If you feel like you're just too old, pray God would change the way you see yourself. God is the one who placed those dreams on your heart, and he will be the one to help you achieve them. With God, all things are possible, and he wants you to realize the dreams he prepared for you.

Take time today to meditate on the dreams you may have given up on, thinking you were too old. Commit to cover those dreams in prayer until they are realized. I want you to say this out loud today and every day until you believe it, "It's not too late, and I'm not too old."

prayer:

Dear Lord, What dreams do you have for me that I've abandoned? Please make my calling clear and show me the path forward. I want to follow your lead and pursue the callings you have for me. I'm excited about my future with you, God. In Jesus' name. Amen.

sassy suggestions:

» Write out a list of dreams you've had throughout your life. Some of them might be funny like the time when you were five and said you wanted to be a Disney princess and skate in the Ice Capades. You probably have to let that one go, but I bet there are several dreams on your list that are still attainable.

» Pray over your list of dreams, asking God to reveal what callings he might have on your life now, for this season.

» Share your dream list with your inner circle and encourage your friends to make their own lists. Cheer each other on as you start chasing your dreams.

» Why not create a dream board to keep your vision in front of you? Write your dreams on a sheet of cardboard and cut out pictures from magazines that reflect your dream. Use stickers, glitter, and markers to decorate your dream board and add inspirational quotes and scripture verses. Once you're finished, place your dream board in a spot you'll see every day.

48

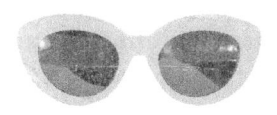

The eyes of the LORD are upon the righteous, and his ears are open unto their cry (Psalm 34:15 KJV).

he notices

Cynthia A. Lovely

There may be times as the years add up and our lives continue to change, we start to feel unimportant or no longer needed. We may have a lifetime of experience behind us and often wisdom to share, but we're not sure if anyone is truly interested. Younger people may act like we don't understand life and our thoughts or input are no longer relevant. Ouch. It may be true that age brings changes and some of them we must learn how to work with or work around. Yet it is hard to combat the attitudes of the young and perky generation coming up behind us.

I admit I may tire out quicker and my physical strength isn't what it used to be when I was younger. This should not stop me from moving forward regardless of the opinion of others. But it still stings. None of us want to feel unnoticed, inferior, or no longer needed. We may fade into the background and slink off into our lonely corner, feeling very neglected, and wondering if anyone even sees us anymore. Instead of sinking into a sad pity party, it is probably time to concentrate on the good news that the Lord God Almighty, who created us, who created all things, he notices us. What a relief to know the One who truly matters, sees us and hears us.

I'm learning to wrap my mind around this scripture and this fact as I go throughout my days, sometimes struggling with a tumult of emotions. Though, I always laugh when I'm feeling invisible and I get one of those cheerful messages in my email inbox: Ten people noticed you today. When the words pop up in my latest email, they always get my attention. My first thought is *Well, at least someone is noticing me, even if it is only on my LinkedIn account.* If you are a member, you probably get the same notifications. It always causes me to wonder who is checking me out.

It is a good feeling to be *noticed* even if it is by a stranger wandering around on social media. With further research, we may find out the notification is someone trying to link up to promote their own business or agenda. Oh well, so much for the thought someone cared enough to notice us. They were only trying to broadcast their business or product. That can be disappointing. Or it may be an old friend who caught our name coming through the social media network. At least that one is a bit more special and may lead us to a re-connection. Either way, the thrill wears off quickly and we move on, hoping to be noticed in our real offline life.

I am thankful we are noticed every day by our heavenly Father. We are never far from his thoughts. Scripture teaches us his eyes are on the righteous. If we are sincerely following the ways of God and trying to live righteously before him, he sees us. He watches us and he notices us. What a beautiful thought. And he not only sees us, but his ears are open and attentive to our cry. *Lord, I feel like no one sees me anymore.* He sees us with his eyes. *God, I am crying out to you today. I desperately need your attention. I don't know the answers, but I know you do.* He hears our voice with his ears. He is not an unseeing, unhearing, unconnected God. No, he is a loving, merciful father who loves us with an everlasting love. No matter who or what is happening around us, God notices us at every age and in every situation. As we recognize this fact and walk in this truth, others may, in turn, notice us and be drawn to the light of God within us.

prayer:

Dear Lord, thank you for noticing me. I am so grateful you see me and you hear me. It is amazing the magnificent God of the universe notices me every day. I pray I will remember this fact, especially as the years climb higher and I may feel unnoticed by others. In Jesus' name. Amen.

sassy suggestions:

» Research scriptures on the word *noticed*. Write out the different meanings and descriptions as they apply to each scripture.

» Begin paying attention to the world around you each day. What do you notice? Are you aware of the people around you daily? Have you been missing someone right in front of you?

» Among your circle of friends and co-workers, who is someone that is usually noticed and who seems to blend in the background. Sometimes the loudest person is always heard, but the quiet one may blend into the walls. Find the unnoticed one and reach out to them.

» As you relate to people, try to focus on your individual conversations and be sure the other person feels noticed by you. Don't be distracted in your conversation. There is nothing worse than sharing your heart with someone and realizing their attention is distracted by everything around them.

» Journal the moments during your day or week when you knew God was noticing you and you understood his care and love for you in each situation. This exercise is sure to leave you with a thankful heart as you are reminded of God's continual care and attention.

49

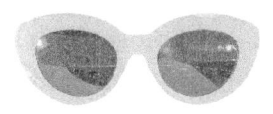

Rejoice in that day and leap for joy, because great is your reward in heaven. For that is how their ancestors treated the prophets (Luke 6:23 NIV).

lifetime achievements

Michelle Medlock Adams

I've been thinking a lot lately about legacy. It's been on my mind ever since this past summer when my buddy and amazing writer Eva Marie Everson was awarded a lifetime achievement award by a prestigious writing and speaking organization that we both belong to—so awesome. As the presenter read over her list of achievements, I was in awe. Not only has she written an extensive and impactful body of work over the course of her life, but also she founded Word Weavers, which continues to grow and minister to writers all over the world. She also runs one of the best writer's conferences in the Christian writing world, the Florida Christian Writers Conference. And that's only to name a few of her notable achievements.

All this got me thinking—no wonder they call them *lifetime achievement* awards, because it takes a lifetime to accomplish all those amazing feats. That's not to say that you can't impact the world when you're young—you absolutely can, and hopefully, we all did. But a lifetime achievement award requires more time.

It's not just about work and accolades. It's not for fame and fortune. A lifetime achievement is the culmination of notable successes. I'd be willing to bet you've collected quite a few of those. Your notable successes might be bringing up kind and brilliant children, caring for an ailing family member, serving in a ministry, preaching the truth in the face of hostility, or giving generously to a noble cause.

The hard truth is that these notable successes aren't always accomplishments that earn plaques or medals. Your lifetime achievement may feel unrecognized. Often, we don't even see the results of our efforts. Maybe you even feel like you've done a whole lot of work for nothing in return. There are no certificates, no banners bearing your name, no spotlights, and no award announcers.

Friend, if you will, please let me be the one to award you with a lifetime achievement award. I don't have a trophy or anything to send you, although I would if I could. But perhaps, for today, this is enough—You've done a great job. You've accomplished so much. And I know you will continue to do great things.

But with all that said, the lifetime achievement award I can offer you isn't the most valuable one to earn. The praises you receive on earth are fun, sure, but they're temporary. We can't take medals and plaques with us, in the end. Not even Nobel Peace Prizes and Olympic medals are worth too much in heaven. The rewards we will receive in heaven don't depend on an impressive resume or peak physical performance. God's rewards are given for withstanding the trials of this world and holding firm in your faith. They are for giving and serving generously and expecting nothing in return. Rewards for stewarding what you've been given. For serving Jesus' people, and in so doing, serving Jesus himself.

A lifetime achievement is really the culmination of all of those successes. It's a collage of all the heart prints we have left along the way. It comes with experience and years and, yes, the wisdom that comes with getting older.

With a lifetime under your belt, you undoubtedly have a lot of wonderful accomplishments. And there's still time. Enjoy the rewards you've received throughout your life and look forward to those waiting for you in heaven. Maybe you feel unnoticed or unappreciated now, but that will all change when you get to heaven and hear, "Well done, my good and faithful servant."

prayer:

Lord, thank you for the rewards you have promised in heaven for those who follow you. And thank you for allowing me to make a difference here on earth. Help me not to rest on my laurels, but rather do more in the years to come. Use me, Lord. I want to continue building my heavenly resume for you.
In Jesus' name. Amen.

sassy suggestions:

» Think back to the successes you've had throughout your life. Create a list and reflect on which achievements are most meaningful to you.

» Gather some friends for an awards ceremony. Have each guest create certificates for everyone in the group. Then, bring out the ceremony snacks and ask everyone to stand up and announce the awards they're presenting. They can be as serious or as silly as you'd like. Some fun ideas could include "Raised 5 Kids and Survived", "World's Best Listener", or "Perfected an Award-Winning Casserole."

50

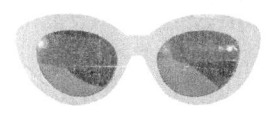

So God created man in His own image, in the image and likeness of God He created him; male and female He created them (Genesis 1:27 AMP).

if you need me, i'll be in the antique store

Connie Clyburn

a visit to the antique/junk stores these days has me feeling a little out of date. I found all the toys I played with as a kid, those plastic bowls and storage containers my mom bought at home parties, even the old tape recorders I remember being so excited to get one year at Christmas. All now considered vintage, some even considered obsolete.

An old doll peering from the top of a towering shelf, once serving as the special guest at a pretend tea party, now wears a faded price tag and a thick veil of dusty cobwebs. If she could talk, she might plead to passersby to give her a chance to be a little girl's best friend again. A rusty tin bread keeper sits on another shelf. I wonder if anyone still uses a bread keeper. Am I as obsolete as some of these vintage pieces? I'll admit I'm no spring chicken, but I know a few facts about life. I think no longer being a spring chicken means I'm not a young chick running around the barnyard anymore. It doesn't mean I'm no longer useful, quite the contrary. I choose to see myself as a treasure.

Those cast-offs in the antique store may appear to be out of date and no longer useful, but many of them bring enormous prices because they are rare. Rare finds are valuable. While the mainstream shopper may overlook such treasures, not realizing what's in front of them, a collector has studied the item inside and out. The collector knows the intricacies of objects and searches them out.

I'm a rare find who is valuable to God, who made me in his image. That makes me sit up straighter and value my worth. Others may not always see my worth, especially as I climb the age ladder, but God does.

It's easy to lose sight of who we are throughout our lives. The world values youth but seems to cast aside those it considers no longer strong and relevant. I beg to differ. God's Word says we are valued players in this game of life. We're still able and capable of making a difference by encouraging others, lending a hand, rallying a cause near and dear to our hearts, or offering ideas to help solve some of today's dilemmas that the years of living have afforded us.

Even if you're feeling a little down from the increasing number of candles on your birthday cake, take heart. What do the *statistics* know? They're not the boss of you. Age simply means a chance to experience something new. It's not the time to get up on a shelf and sit out for the rest of life. Get out of that slump, get out of the house, and into life. God has much for us to accomplish and it doesn't stop at a certain age. I intend to keep on giving, doing, and going. I have too many ideas that I haven't even started on—no time to quit now. It's go time.

prayer:

Dear Lord, Thank you for loving and valuing me all the days of my life, even on the days when I don't see value in myself. Help me see myself through your eyes. You have created me for a purpose, and I intend to accomplish all you have for me to do, as you work through me, causing me to triumph over every false identity the world tries to lay on me. You, Lord, are my strength and my shield. I love you.
In Jesus' name. Amen.

sassy suggestions:

» **Find yourself in God's Word. These verses will help you get started.**
   Song of Solomon 4:7 (AMP)
   2 Corinthians 5:17 (AMP)
   Ephesians 2:10 (AMP)

» **You are relevant and your years of living have given you experience to share with those around you.** Maybe a young mother could use a bit of advice about raising her kids in today's world. Times have changed, but kids are still little humans going through the same stages of growth as generations before them. A newly married couple experiencing relationship ups and downs might benefit from tips on navigating rough patches.

» **Renewed and refreshed.** Our mindset has so much to do with how we see ourselves as we age. Allow God to renew your mind according to Romans 12:2 (AMP)

» **Charged and ready. Psalm 103:5 (AMP).**

» **A spa day may be just what you need.** No money or time for a professional spa? No problem. Turn your own bathroom into an oasis with rose petals floating on a warm bath, scented candles casting a soft glow and decadent chocolates waiting tub side.

51

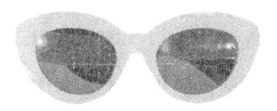

Their children will be mighty in the land; the generation of the upright will be blessed (Psalm 112:2 NIV).

legacy of love

Michelle Medlock Adams

As I held my mother's hand during the last moments of her life, I noticed my hands looked exactly like hers.

I have my mother's hands, I thought. *I wish I had my mother's ability to love.*

Mom had such a special way of making everyone feel loved. I always felt like I was Mom's favorite child, but if you asked my sister and brother, "Who was Mom's favorite?" they'd each point to themselves. She bought me *just because* presents throughout the year. She baked her special chocolate oatmeal cookies whenever I needed a little cheering up. And she made up funny little songs to fit whatever situation I might go through. You just couldn't be in a bad mood when you were with my Mom. Her love would bubble out of her and onto you, and before long; you would be singing one of her silly songs, too. Truly, her capacity to love her family, her friends, her community, and her church was quite inspiring.

After Mom went to heaven on May 3, 2006, I felt the immense weight of that loss. Not only had I lost my best friend and my #1 cheerleader, but also, I had lost the greatest example of walking in love, faith, and hope that I'd ever known.

That's when I had a realization. Her just because gifts, chocolate oatmeal cookies, and silly little songs didn't have to end with her. Her ability to make everyone feel special did not have to die with Mom. After decades of my mother showering me with her love, and living a life of extravagant love, I could choose to either let it go or take up that mantle myself.

I realized it was my turn.

So I started giving just because presents to my daughters. I started baking them Mamaw's special chocolate oatmeal cookies. I started making up silly little songs about life.

Why? Because I wanted to create those same wonderful memories of love and laughter with my daughters. Mom left a legacy of love, and I was determined to keep it alive with my girls. I still am. Plus, now I get to share that extravagant love with my six grandchildren, making each one think he/she is my favorite.

How about you? Are you leaving a legacy?

Take a look at the actions and attitudes you have passed along to your children. Notice the impact you have on the people around you with each interaction. Consider how the world is a different place because you have been here. How do you think you will be remembered?

If pondering that question has left you feeling anxious or sad, don't worry. It's not too late to make an impact. You still have time to leave a legacy.

It's no wonder we spend so much time thinking about legacy. The Bible puts a lot of emphasis on the idea of passing on a legacy of love and faith. Ever since Adam and Eve had their first children, passing a legacy from generation to generation has been hard-wired into us. We've been charged with passing the wisdom and love of God to the next generation.

The lessons you've learned, the prayers you've prayed, the feelings you inspire in others, and what you've created are all parts of your legacy. You can pass your legacy down in many different forms. Perhaps it's the lessons you've imparted to your family, the love you've planted in the hearts of the people you see every day, the actions you've taken to give your family a better life, or a career that has made the world a better place. Even the smallest actions can make a lasting impact.

Take a moment to ask yourself what heart imprints will you leave on this world? Ask the Lord to help you build a legacy of love today that will continue long after you are gone.

prayer:

Dear Lord, Please help me build a legacy of love, especially for my family. I want to leave the world a better, more hope-filled place than I found it. Please use me in this season of my life for something that will last longer than my own life—something greater than myself. Lord, fill me up with your love so that I can let it bubble out of me everywhere I go. In Jesus' name. Amen.

sassy suggestions:

» **Recipes for Life.** If you're an old school cook, you probably don't know how many pinches of oregano you put in your meatballs, but you may want to figure it out so you can pass down your recipes to your loved ones. That way, they can recreate your famous food once you've moved to heaven. Spend a day in the kitchen with your children or your grandchildren and write down your most-prized recipes. Do the same with your other older relatives and put together a family recipe book.

» **Research and Rejoice.** You may not be a history buff, but your family's history is quite important and fun to research. Why not make it your family project to discover something new about your family's history and document it?

» **Precious Artifacts.** Some say young people just don't appreciate antiques anymore, but that's not entirely true. It's not that they don't care about family heirlooms, the next generation just doesn't want boxes of meaningless stuff stored in their attics. Create a scrapbook with photos of your life's artifacts—family heirlooms, personal treasures, and important objects—and write the meaning of those pieces beside each one. You might find your family takes far more interest in using the items you pass down to them if there is a story attached to each item.

52

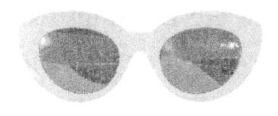

For you are a holy people (set apart) to the Lord your God; and the Lord has chosen you out of all the peoples who are on the earth to be a people for his own possession.
Deuteronomy 14:2 (AMP).

we are his treasure

Connie Clyburn

a quote I've heard many times recently resonated with me, "To the world you're one in four trillion, but to God you are a one and only."

I let it sink into my mind that often fails to see my own worth. In a world full of millions of people, I am a "one and only." I'm an only child, so I can relate to that. My parents celebrated me on every occasion—no birthday went unnoticed, every Christmas celebrated with most everything for which I asked. Easters had mom making a big basket full of candy and surprises.

God loves and adores me even more. He houses his own spirit within me like a prized vessel full of rare, expensive oil. I am his treasure. So are you.

He created his treasure for a reason—not to hide us away in some uncharted territory for someone with a faded map to find later, but for good works. We are running this race on purpose from beginning to end. I know sometimes it can feel like life has served its purpose. The kids are grown and out on their own. Working as a valued member of a team is a distant memory played out in photos of your retirement party. Perhaps your parents are gone and all it seems you have left are precious memories to treasure.

When God created you, he set your own special life before you to live. You are here for a specific purpose, to fill a unique role. There are stories of people well into their 90s and even past 100 doing astounding feats, running their course, and making a difference in their communities. Stories like that inspire because those individuals didn't see age as an obstacle. Instead, they used it as a trampoline to propel them into their next adventure.

I'm reminded of a gentleman at my church I saw as such a treasure. Horace's bright smile, hearty "hello" and firm handshake welcomed church members and visitors through the building's front door for years—well into his 90s. It was Horace's job. That is what God had him doing, after he had worked hard for years, loving Inez, his wife, and raising their family with her. I still think of Horace often and miss him. He left an impression I'll never forget. That and the baby smooth skin he attributed to the Vaseline he applied to his face each night.

I will honor Horace's memory by being relevant and active in older age. I want to hold my own in push-up contests when challenged by the younger generation. Well, maybe not push-ups, but I want to hold my own and still be contributing somehow.

We are created in Christ Jesus for good works. It doesn't say big works or expensive works—just good works. A good life full of good works is ahead whether you're 15 or 50, 19 or 90. Age, as they say, is truly a number. And if age counts at all, it is significant for planning birthday parties, for making precious memories, for raising families and holding grandchildren, and for counting the ways in which you love someone.

Our years are for making the most of every moment God gives us. Every day, we can get up and share the treasure that is within us. There's so much still to do. We can enrich other's lives in little ways and even with magnificent acts of kindness. When we do that, our own lives will be enriched. A successful life is not always scaling great heights or having our names in headlines. It is found in the little tasks we do every day. That is what makes our lives significant until the last drop is used up. It happens when we share the treasure that we are.

prayer:

Dear Lord, Thank you for treasuring me. Thank you for health and joy. I ask you to help me continue to see my purpose whatever my stage in life. I want to live a life pleasing to you. Help me share the precious bounty you've placed in me. I love you. Thank you.
In Jesus' name. Amen.

sassy suggestions:

» **Send a Card.** Make someone else feel like a treasure. Pick out a few special cards to keep on hand for sending to friends.

» **Make a call.** A quick call to check in means a mint to those who don't get out and have few visitors, and it will help them feel special. A surprise call can brighten an otherwise dull, uneventful day for both of you.

» **Run an errand.** Know someone who doesn't drive or perhaps you have a friend who's sick and unable to get out for a few days? Have them give you their grocery list and then make a quick delivery. You'll not only be helping, but it will also be a big stress reducer for them too.

» **Bake a cake.** Keep a cake mix and frosting on hand to whip up a treat for a friend, loved one, or neighbor quickly. Decorate it with colored sugar sprinkles, wrap it up with a bow, and drop it off. Voila! You've brightened up another day and made a valuable connection.

» **Give a gift.** If you love making crafts, visit your local craft store's clearance aisle for fun ideas to create homemade gifts to give. Who doesn't enjoy giving and getting gifts? It's always a win-win when you take time to share your talents with others. What seems small to you may be a big deal to someone else

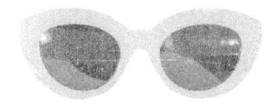

acknowledgments

Thank you to Bold Vision Books for believing in this project! I'm grateful for this opportunity.

My wonderful co-authors, Michelle and Cynthia – thank you for allowing me to write this book with you. The best is yet to come!

—Connie

Thank you to Bold Vision for taking on this fun project. And to my writing mentors, friends and family who help on this writing journey. Thanks to my fab co-authors and thank you Michelle, for including us on this grand adventure. Special thanks to my dear husband, Dwayne, for being my biggest fan, support, and encouragement through it all. To God be the glory!

—Cynthia

Thank you, Rhonda Rhea, for championing this book from Day 1. You're the best! And, special thanks to my buddies and coauthors Connie and Cynthia for being my friends through every season. Also, I want to thank my husband, Jeff, who has been my biggest cheerleader and best friend for more than 30 years. And, lastly, I want to thank my Heavenly Father for allowing me to continue writing for Him. I am blessed.

—Michelle

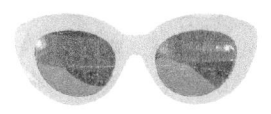

about the authors

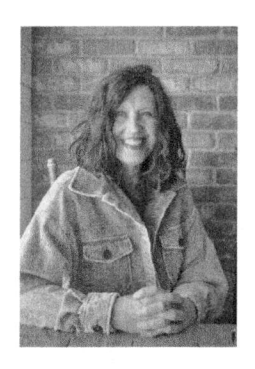

Connie Clyburn has been known to climb a mountainside for a story. It's true! Her writing career began as a newspaper reporter in her native East Tennessee, before traveling into the coal country of Kentucky to work at weekly newspapers there. Soon enough, her dream of authoring books came true with the release of her first children's book, *Willy the Silly-Haired Snowman's Great Adventure*. She also coauthored the e-devotional, *Peace and Promise During a Crisis*.

Her ability to see the "funny" in most every situation led her to develop her brand, *Wisdom from the Doublewide*. You'll most likely find Connie, with coffee in hand and cowboy boots on her feet, writing in her home office, Tenasi Road Studio, or enjoying laughs and good food with close friends at a favorite restaurant. She also enjoys using her amateur detective skills to help the heroine solve a mystery in the latest whodunit movie - when she's not out chasing sunsets.

She is also an award-winning writer whose articles have appeared in newspapers, magazines and on the web. Read about her musings on life through her blog featured on the website, Wisdom from the Doublewide.

You can connect with her on social media here:

Facebook: https://www.facebook.com/p/Connie-Clyburn-WriterAuthor-100065641743351/ and at https://www.facebook.com/connie.clyburn
Instagram: @wisdomfromthedoublewide
Twitter: @connieclyburn
Pinterest: Connie Clyburn
LinkedIn: Connie Clyburn

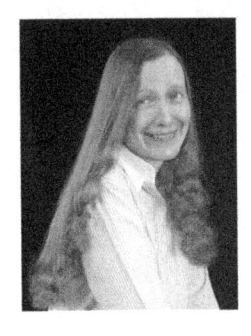

If you place **Cynthia A. Lovely** by the ocean, a lake, on the sound or bayside, she will end up writing all day. Something about being near a beautiful body of water inspires and energizes her. This inspiration has resulted in over sixty articles and stories in magazines, newspapers, and anthologies including several Chicken Soup for the Soul books.

Her Christmas stories generated book signings in Saratoga Springs, as part of Victorian Street Walk where she enjoyed dressing in full Victorian attire. She also signed books at Inn Victoria in Chester, Vermont with a surprise interview and article in the *Vermont Journal*. But the best experience was a story from *My Amazing Mom* with a full article in the *Gazette* honoring her precious mother on Mother's Day.

Cynthia loves words! She lives in the country and finds ideas all around her from the fox chasing a rooster down her walkway to surviving fierce winter storms with over 3 feet of snow. She is co-author of the devotional e-book, *Peace and Promise During a Crisis* and has written for *Pandemic Moments* by Yvonne Lehman. Stepping out of her comfort zone, she accepted and now enjoys speaking engagements with women's groups and even a writing workshop at the local library.

If not sitting by the water, she may be found playing piano/sax duets with her husband, creating theme songs for the latest church musical, or facing the challenges of being a minister's wife, in upstate New York. She is an avid reader, writer, and musician and is forever grateful for the God-gift of her husband, along with the gain of a "lovely" signature.

www.cynthiaalovely.com

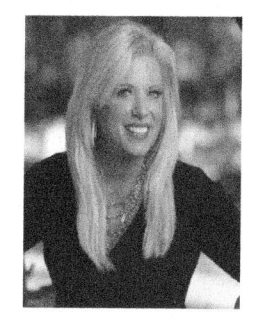

Michelle Medlock Adams is a New York Times best-selling ghostwriter and an award-winning journalist, earning top honors from the Associated Press, the Society of Professional Journalists, and the Hoosier State Press Association to name a few.

Author of over 100 books with over 3 million books sold, Michelle has won more than 90 industry awards for her own journalistic endeavors, including the prestigious Golden Scroll for Best Children's Book in 2023, 2022, 2021, 2020, 2019 and 2018 for *Our God is Bigger Than That!*, *Dachshund Through the Snow*, *Cuddle-Up Prayers*, *How Much Does God Love You?*, *Dinosaur Devotions*, and *My First Day of School*. And, over the past three years, she has added several first-place honors from the Christian Market Book Awards, the Selah Book Awards, the Moonbeam Children's Book Awards, and the Illumination Book Awards in multiple categories.

Since graduating with a journalism degree from Indiana University, Michelle has written more than 1,700 articles for newspapers, magazines, and websites; acted as a stringer for the Associated Press; written for a worldwide ministry; hosted "Joy In Our Town" TV show for the Trinity Broadcasting Network; blogged twice weekly for Guideposts; written a weekly column for a Midwest newspaper; founded and served as president of Platinum Literary Services; and served as an adjunct professor at Taylor University. Today, she is Chairman of the Board of Advisors for Serious Writer, Inc.; owner and editor of her very own children's book imprint "Wren & Bear Books"—a division of End Game Press; and a much sought-after speaker at professional writing conferences and women's retreats all over the United States. When not working on her own assignments, Michelle ghostwrites articles, blog posts, and books for celebrities, politicians, and some of today's most effective and popular ministers.

Michelle is celebrating her recent releases: *Love Connects Us All*, *Springtime For Your Spirit*, *Our God is Bigger Than That!*, and *Fly High*.

Michelle is married to her high school sweetheart, Jeff, and they have two daughters, Abby and Allyson, two sons-in-law, and six adorable grandchildren. She and Jeff share their home in Southern Indiana with two diva dachshunds, a rescue Poodle/Shepherd mix, and two spoiled kitties. When not writing or teaching writing, Michelle enjoys bass fishing, cheering on Indiana University sports teams, watching Doris Day movies, and all things leopard print.

http://www.michellemedlockadams.com/

Made in the USA
Middletown, DE
24 July 2024